Indigenous Health:
The Intersectionality of History, Social Justice, and Equity

Indigenous Health:
The Intersectionality of History, Social Justice, and Equity

AUTHORS:
AUSTIN MARDON
KOLBY HOARE
ROKYA HARUN
MARIA ASHRAF
HAFSA BINTE YOUNUS
MICHAEL OWANGA
RYAN DOLEWEERD
BRIANNA BEDRAN
CHRISTINA MACDONALD
RIDA KHAN
RAZAN AHMED

EDITOR
CATHERINE MARDON

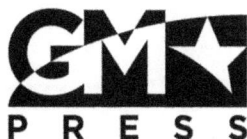

GM★
P R E S S

First Printing: 2023

Typeset and Cover Design by Josh Harnack & Monette Rockliff
ISBN: 978-1-77889-061-1
eBook ISBN: 978-1-77889-062-8

Golden Meteorite Press
103 11919 82 St NW
Edmonton, AB T5B 2W3
www.goldenmeteoritepress.com

TABLE OF CONTENTS

CHAPTER 1: KEY LEGISLATIVE MOMENTS FOR INDIGENOUS PEOPLES IN CANADA AND IMPACTS *(Kolby Hoare)* 10

CHAPTER 2: ENVIRONMENTAL RACISM AND ITS ASSOCIATED SOCIAL, POLITICAL AND HEALTH CONCERS FOR INDIGENOUS PEOPLE IN CANADA *(Rokya Harun)* 22

CHAPTER 3: ISSUES IN ACCESS TO AND PROVISION OF HEALTHCARE FOR INDIGENOUS PEOPLE IN CANADA *(Maria Ashraf)* 33

CHAPTER 4: MENTAL HEALTH AND ITS ASSOCIATED CONCERNS IN INDIGENOUS PEOPLE *(Hafsa Binte Younus)* 45

CHAPTER 5: INTERGENERATIONAL TRAUMA AND THE EFFECTS OF RESIDENTIAL SCHOOLS ON INDIGENOUS PEOPLE IN CANADA TODAY *(Michael Owanga)* 57

CHAPTER 6: THE ROLES AND RELATIONSHIPS BETWEEN ANIMALS AND INDIGENOUS PEOPLE *(Ryan Doleweerd)* 67

CHAPTER 7 GENDERED IMPACTS: VIOLENCE AND IDENTITY ERASURE AGAINST INDIGENOUS WOMEN AND GIRL'S IN CANADA AND THE U.S *(Brianna Bedran)* 78

CHAPTER 8 : RESPECTING INDIGENOUS PEOPLES AS A NON-INDIGENOUS PERSON: EXPLORING ALLYSHIP AND INTERSECTIONALITY FROM THE PERSPECTIVE OF AN ALLY *(Christina MacDonald)* 89

CHAPTER 9 EXPLORING THE OVERREPRESENTATION OF INDIGENOUS CHILDREN IN FOSTER CARE *(Rida Khan)* 102

CHAPTER 10 THE EDUCATION GAP IN INDIGENOUS COMMUNITIES *(Razan Ahmed)* 114

INTRODUCTION

Indigenous communities lived, explored, and searched Canada ever before the settlers arrived. As the time passed by, they faced several barriers from legislation, treaties, and even in today's ociety. Throughout the chapters, we will explore various perspectives and issues that are present in indigenous communities and some of the allyship methods.

In Chapter 1, we will explore events such as the Red Dress Project and Every Child Matters movements. We will talk about what caused these events. The answer lies in observing keylegislative movements by the British Monarch, and the subsequent Canadian government. This observation will illustrate a relationship founded on mutual respect and cooperation, and its evolution to subjugation and forgotten sentiments, with legislation serving as a colonial tool to legitimise their capricious behaviour.

In Chapter 2, we will analyse environmental impacts. Marginalised groups and Indigenouscommunities in particular are subject to living in environmental conditions that would not be acceptable for other groups in Canada.

In Chapter 3, this chapter focuses on indigenous health and healthcare in the light of access and provision. It seeks to answer questions about how indigenous health is approached in Canada. What are the barriers to access and provision and what are the possible solutions?

In Chapter 4, we research the mental health concerns in the Indeginous people. It talks about the factors that lead to mental health concern in these communities. It also discusses the common mental health concerns and some of the barriers faced by these communities.

In Chapter 5, the chapter focuses on intergenerational trauma and effects of residential schools. This chapter focuses on past legislation and policies that directly affected Indigenous Canadians in the past and the impacts that they have had on their descendants today. The concept of intergenerational trauma is explained in the context of how Indigenous Canadians are currently experiencing it as a result of The Indian Act, residential schools, and the Sixties Scoop.

In Chapter 6, this chapter will explore the roles of animals in the lives of Indigneous people from around the world, both past and present. In this line of investigation, one will learn about how the lives of Indigenous people and the animals in their own respective regions are intertwined, and as a result will understand why the Indigenous people value the importance of a good relationship with animals.

In Chapter 7, we will be exploring the gendered impacts of colonisation on marginalised Indigenous women and girls. While colonisation is often described as a problem of the past, the impacts are long lasting and are perpetuated by existing structural factors that include legislations, negligence of the criminal justice system, and socioeconomic factors that work against their favour.

In Chapter 8, written from the perspective of a non-Indigenous person, this chapter aims to show respect for Indigenous Peoples by exploring resources that currently exist for non-Indigenous individuals to better understand what it means to be an ally. By delving into the concepts of allyship and intersectionality, this chapter aims to mobilise knowledge for those who want to learn more about being an ally but may not know where to start.

In Chapter 9, we will investigate respecting Indigenous Peoples as a non-Indigenous person: Exploring allyship and intersectionality from the perspective of an ally. The Canadian Child Welfare system has clear overrepresentation of Indigenous youth due to the discriminatory biases shown by child welfare workers. This leads to detrimental and differential impact on Indigenous youth.

In Chapter 10, we will address the education gap in indigenous communities. Canada has a concerning Indigenous Education Gap—a disparity in educational achievement between Indigenous and non-Indigenous people. The Indigenous Education Gap is widening and rising quickly across Canada. Bridging the education gap is thus a critical component of any plan for enhancing the prosperity, health, and well-being of Canada's indigenous population, as well as eliminating marginalisation.

CHAPTER 1

KEY LEGISLATIVE MOMENTS FOR INDIGENOUS PEOPLES IN CANADA AND IMPACTS

By Kolby Hoare

INTRODUCTION

Recent events such as the Red Dress Project, and Every Child Matters Movement have shed light on the unsettling realities faced by Indigneous peoples in Canada, and horrified many Canadians. As we seek to better understand these realities Canadians may ask themselves how such egregious and discriminatory acts could be legally facilitated against Indigenous peoples. The answer lies in observing key legislative movements by the British Monarch, and the subsequent Canadian government. This observation will illustrate a relationship founded on mutual respect and cooperation, and its evolution to subjugation and forgotten sentiments, with legislation serving as a colonial tool to legitimise their capricious behaviour.

Truth and Reconciliation - a concept once unknown in Canada, has become commonplace in the national dialogue. Hundreds of years of mistreatment towards Indigenous[1] peoples led to a reality that could no longer be ignored. While Canadians continue to learn these truths they may wonder how Canada-Indigenous relations ever became so unjust and discriminatory. Indigenous issues in Canada are complex, multifaceted, and intertwined in many ways.

---

1   'In this chapter the term Indigenous is used to refer to First Nations (status and non-status), Métis and Inuit, as acollective group. When Indigenous is used to describe the subjects of legislation and discrimination one must note that some particular practices of this discrimination may only be applicable to particular members of the collective, such as status, or First Nations individuals. Additionally, the term Indigenous has been chosen over Aboriginal to indicate Indigenous peoples international legal rights under the United Nations Declaration of the Rights of Indigenous Peoples.

However, it is pivotal to acknowledge and understand the role that key historical and legislative moments have played in systematically exploiting and suppressing Indigenous peoples in Canada. Thus, the aim of this chapter is to highlight select historical and legislative events that have led to the manifestation of Indigenous conditions we have come to know in Canada today. It is important to note that this chapter is only to inform readers on a rudimentary level, and further, more profound reading on the subject matter is encouraged.

THE ROYAL PROCLAMATION OF 1763

While there is a long history of colonial-First Nations relations in North America preceding the Royal Proclamation of 1763, we will start our understanding of Canadian-Indigenous relations with this historical document as it largely laid the groundwork for what would subsequently become British (Canada)-Indigenous relations. In a reductionist simplification, the Seven Years War was a battle primarily between Britain and France (amongst others), over colonial expansion and conquest in North America (and elsewhere). During the war, both Britain and France had a series of alliances with different First Nations groups who fought alongside them in their North American battles and were of great service to their military efforts. At the conclusion of the war, the British emerged victorious. This resulted in Britain acquiring North American land concessions from France as part of the 1763 Treaty of Paris. After the acquisition, King George III of Britain issued a Royal Proclamation. In its essence the proclamation stated the Monarch's administrative right over territory and colonies in North America. This declaration established British jurisdiction, and incorporated large swaths of North American territory into the rule of British parliamentary institutions – including much land inhabited by First Nations, which would later become Canada.

The Royal Proclamation also addressed First Nations rights and relations with the Monarchy and its North American colonies. These relations were incredibly important to the Monarchy at the time as First Nations groups continued warring with the British following the conclusion of the Seven Years War. During this continued warring, First Nations groups had successfully taken multiple British forts within the interior lands, and were actively taking on others (Hele, 2021). Thus, in the eyes of the Monarchy, their undefined relations with First Nations peoples posed a large insecurity to creating sustained peace in the region, and ultimately their continued success in North America colonial ventures.

There are two main implications stemming from the proclamation that are important to recognize. The first of these implications is the delineation of Indigenous rights and territories in North America, according to the Monarchy. The proclamation stated that lands outside of the delineated jurisdiction of the colonies, or the Hudson's Bay Company, and lands west of said colonies were strictly forbidden by colonial peoples for purchase, settlement or possession without the leave or license of the British Monarchy.

And whereas it is just and reasonable, and essential to Our Interest and the Security of Our Colonies, that the several Nations or Tribes of Indians, with whom We are connected, and who live under Our Protection, should not be molested or disturbed in the Possession of such Parts of Our Dominions and Territories as, not having been ceded to, or purchased by Us, are reserved to them, or any of them, as their Hunting Grounds.(Royal Proclamation, 1763)

However, in time, the Royal Proclamation of 1763 would prove to be a double-edged sword. While it did indeed represent rights and protections for First Nations peoples, it gave the British Monarchy exclusive jurisdiction over all future negotiations with First Nations peoples. Additionally, the proclamation assumed First Nations peoples were residing within the dominions and territories of the Monarchy. Thus, any change of lands between First Nations and colonies would do so under the facilitation of the Monarchy, with the utilization of Indian Affairs. This led to the foundation of the treaty making process between Indigenous peoples and the Monarchy, a practice that would eventually evolve and take place between Indigenous peoples and the government of Canada, (Crown-Indigenous Relations and Northern Affairs Canada, 2016).

Following the Royal Proclamation, the Monarchy instructed Sir William Johnson, superintendent of Indian affairs for the northern colonies to make peace with the interior or western First Nations and gather support for the new proclamation. To do so Sir William Johnson created a treaty with approximately 24 First Nations, referred to as the 1764 Treaty of Niagara. To conclude this treaty several agreements and concessions were made. The First Nations involved conceded to return British prisoners, and to cease contact with Britain's enemies (especially France), and accept the terms of the proclamation. In return Britain promised to compensate First Nations trader's losses resulting from the 1763 conflict, authorize First Nations passage across the Proclamation line, and finally, to prosecute settlers committing crimes against First Nations (Hele, 2021). The First Nations signatories exchanged diplomatic Wampum belts between each other and with Johnson. Johnson's belt depicted two figures holding hands, and symbolized friendship and alliance between the nations and the crown. With hexagons representing council fires – presumably to honor the diplomacy that had just occurred, and future diplomacy to be discussed (Hele, 2021). The First Nations gifted Johnson a two-row Wampum belt said to indicate peace, friendship, and respect (Hele, 2021),

Following the conclusion of the 1764 Treaty of Niagara the first official land treaty was signed.In time different forms of treaties would cover the better part of what would become Canada. However, while First Nations groups agreed to lay down arms and conduct treaties of equality and good faith with the Crown, this good faith, and the sentiments embedded in the Wampum belt would eventually prove unrequited by colonial powers.

CHANGING PERSPECTIVES

Within 50 years of the first land surrenders that brought settlers to Upper Canada, non-First Nations inhabitants surpassed First Nations populations in the Great Lakes basin(Crown-Indigenous Relations and Northern Affairs Canada, 2011). Around the same time the British perception of First Nations peoples was changing with contemporary events. After First Nations peoples fought along the British and played a pivotal role in winning the War of 1812, and peace ensued, the British stopped seeing the strategic military role of First Nations allies.Instead, ideas of British superiority and missionary zeal catalyzed the desire to bring 'civilized' British life to the First Nations peoples in the colonies of Upper and Lower Canada (Crown-Indigenous Relations and Northern Affairs Canada, 2011). As such, the Crown's Indian Department transformed into a medium for the new plan of civilizing First Nations peoples. Often quoting a belief that it was their duty to bring Christianity and new agriculture practice to First Nations peoples (Crown-Indigenous Relations and Northern Affairs Canada, 2011). These initiatives and sentiments can be seen in the fact that the first 'Indian' Residential School in what we now know as Canada was started in 1831 (National Centre for Truth and Reconciliation,n.d.).

CANADIAN CONFEDERATION AND THE INDIAN ACT

Before confederation occurred on July 1st, 1867, there was an appetite for a united Canada amongst the provinces. However, this dream could only be accomplished through expansionist policies, which the Royal Proclamation made difficult. Additionally, with settlers now outnumbering Indigenous peoples, and there no longer a need for their assistance in war, there was little desire on the part of colonial powers to co-govern, or properly accommodate First Nations rights as previously promised in the Royal Proclamation of 1763. Contrarily, as previously mentioned colonial powers in what would soon be Canada wanted to 'civilize' Indigenous peoples and assimilate them towards their goals. As a result, the fifth Parliament of the Province of Canada (formally Upper Canada and Lower Canada) passed what would be called the Gradual Civilization Act in 1857. In the act Indigenous peoples could voluntarily relinquish their treaty rights, in return for a land divided out for homesteading and voting privileges. Ultimately this policy was an abysmal failure and soon Canada would incorporate in 1867, the same year the Indian Act was passed.

At its core the objective of the Indian Act was to "subsume[] a number of colonial laws that aimed to eliminate First Nations culture in favor of assimilation into Euro-Canadian society" (Parrott, 2022, para. 1). However, the Indian Act did not affect all Indigenous peoples in Canada, only those who, according to the government, had obtained "Indian Status" having been "registered Indians." A practice that had long been in the works with agreements such as the 1850 Act for the better protection of the Lands and Property of the Indians in Lower Canada. Which set important criteria for what it meant to be an 'Indian' and helped create precedent for the concept of 'status' (Parrott, 2022). Importantly, "treaty Indians" – Indigenous peoples in Canada who were part of a treaty deal – were also considered registered Indians, and therefore subject to the Indian Act (Statistics Canada, 2021). Therefore, the Indian Act used 'Indian' status as a method to assert power over the Indigenous peoples of Canada. This status was often derived through treaty rights, antithetical to the governmental objectives. Thus, Indigenous peoples who had joined into arrangements of treaties under the contexts of mutual respect, equality, and cooperation now found themselves subject to the legislative jurisdiction of Canada's Parliament who asserted legislative power over "Indians, and Lands reserved for the Indians" (Parrott, 2022).

The Indian Act addressed all Indigenous groups as homogenous and aimed at assimilating them into colonial society. It stifled these groups in fundamental ways. The act prohibited the expression of Indigenous culture within their own governance. It supplanted Indigenous government institutions of hereditary leaders, (or First Nations Chiefs) with band councils and elections, and excluded women from Indigenous politics (Hanson & Crey, 2009). The act also made it illegal for First Nations peoples and their communities to raise funds in the pursuit of land claims (Hanson & Crey, 2009). Regarding cultural expression, the Indian act outlawed Indigenous religious ceremonies, cultural gatherings, potlatch, festivals, dances, powwows and more (Hanson & Crey, 2009). The act also allowed for egregious policies of control over Indigenous peoples. Including the pass system — a process by which First Nations people had to present a travel document authorized by an Indian agent to leave and return to their reserves" (Nestor, 2018). Additionally, the previously failed Gradual Civilization Act of 1876 (as mentioned before) and its follow up Gradual Enfranchisement act both became part of the Indian Act in 1876. The Gradual act gave the Superintendent General of Indian Affairs extreme control over status Indians. It granted them the power to determine who was of moral character and deserve certain benefits, including things such as if a widowed enfranchised Indian could therefore keep her children, and laid the groundwork for the 60s scoop[2] (Hanson & Crey, 2009). The Gradual Enfranchisement Act also severely restricted band councils' power to govern, determined who was eligible for band and treaty benefits. As well as beginning gender-based restrictions to status (Hanson & Crey, 2009). Lastly, the Indian Act laid the legal foundation for the creation and implementation of heinous industrial and residential schools.

Over time some of the rules stemming from the Indian Act were repealed, retreated, or changed. But ultimately ruthless practices deriving their bases from the Indian Act proceeded for a shamefully long time, as exemplified by the closing of the last residential school in 1996. Today it is well known that these acts constituted a genocide on Indigenous people, and have created intergenerational trauma for Indigenous communities.

THE WHITE PAPER OF 1969

By 1969 in light of the civil rights movement in the United States Canadians began to recognize that the relationship between Indigenous peoples in Canada and the government of Canada had degraded to an unacceptable state. Acknowledgment of the many socioeconomic barriers that Indigenous peoples faced led to government consolations with Indigenous peoples. During these consultations Indigenous representatives expressed reoccurring themes of concern. These included "Aboriginal and treaty rights, title to the land, self-determination, and access to education and health care" (Hanson & Crey, 2009, para. 6). Recognizing the terrible state for Indigenous peoples Prime Minister Pierre Trudeau introduced a document now referred to as the White Paper of 1969. The aim of this document was to effectively revoke all legislative matters or special titles for Indigenous peoples, most prominently, the Indian Act. As Trudeau saw it, the Indian Act was a prejudice piece of legislation that gave the Canadian government the means to discriminate against and void Indigenous peoples of their rights

2   The 60s scoop refers to a time in which a large number of Aboriginal children were removed from their families and put into the child welfare system, most often without the consent of the families or bands.

and opportunities. Thus, the white paper aimed to

Eliminate Indian status[,] dissolve the Department of Indian Affairs[,] [a]bolish the Indian Act[,] [c]onvert reserve land to private property that can be sold by the band or its members[,] [t]ransfer responsibility for Indian affairs from the federal government to the province and integrate these services into those provided to other Canadian citizens[,] [p]rovide funding for economic development and appoint a commissioner to address outstanding land claims and gradually terminate existing treaties (Hanson & Crey, 2009, para. 4).

At its core, the white paper would effectively eliminate any differentiation between Indigenous peoples in Canada, and other Canadian citizens.

The White Paper was seen as a tone-deaf proposition that failed to recognize the grievances brought forward by the Indigenous consultation. It did not recognize their treaty rights, or historic grievances – especially pertaining to land rights. On the contrary, the White Paper appeared to be a decisive and final blow to Indigenous rights. A final step in assimilation predicated on alleviating Indigenous peoples of their legitimated suffering at the hands of the government. But Indigenous peoples did not see the white paper as a means of alleviating their discrimination, but excusing the federal government of their obligations to them, causing the rejection of this proposed paper.

THE CONSTITUTION ACT 1982

In 1980 the Trudeau government was looking to patriate Canada from Britain. Part of this process was the creation of what would later become the Constitution Act. The initial constitution proposal made little mention in terms of Indigenous rights, and did not practice consultation with Indigenous representatives. This created concern amongst Indigenous peoples in Canada that their historic rights under the British would be lost in the transfers of powers, and that their right to autonomous decision making would be undermined (Hanson & Crey, 2009). As a result, Indigenous groups in Canada gathered funds and awareness to advocate for their inclusion in the patriation. This included relaying their concerns in front of international audiences, such as the United Nations and the British Parliament (Hanson & Crey, 2009).

Their fight for recognition led to Section 35 being added to the constitution in time for patriation in 1982. Section 35 initially consisted of clauses (1) and (2). Clause one of section 35 recognizes and affirms the treaty rights of Indigenous peoples in Canada Section two, defines Indigenous, (or Aboriginal peoples as referred to in the act) as including "Indian, Inuit and Métis peoples of Canada." Clauses (3) and (4) were subsequently developed in 1983-4 as a result of consultations with Indigenous representatives during the First Ministers' Conference on Indigenous Rights in March of 1983 (Justice Law Website, 2022). Clause three clarifies that *treaty rights* include rights that now exist by way of land claims agreements, or may be so acquired. And clause four mandates that these rights are guaranteed to both men and women (Justice Law Website, 2022). This clause was added after lengthy campaigns by women's groups, who were unrepresented in the initial discussions and experienced systemic gender discrimination from such legislation as Bill C-31.[3] Additionally, Section 25 guarantees that no rights protected under the Charter will be used to abrogate or derogate from rights belonging to Indigenous people (including land rights and rights under the Royal Proclamation). While section 35.1 (a) and (b) state that amendment to this would take place with all First Ministers, the Prime Minister, and the participation and discussion of (as according to the document) Indigenous peoples in this matter.

There are mixed reviews regarding the success of the constitution act on the lives of Indigenous peoples. Some see it as a reinforcement of superiority of colonial laws and beliefs, while others believe it does little to uphold the rights of Indigenous peoples. However, others believe it is a codified and public declaration to ward off further degradation of Indigenous rights in

---

3   "Bill C-31, or a Bill to Amend the Indian Act, passed into law in April 1985 to bring the Indian Act into line with gender equality under the Canadian Charter of Rights and Freedoms. It proposed modifications to various sections of the Indian Act, including significant changes to Indian status and band membership, with three major goals: to address gender discrimination of the Indian Act, to restore Indian status to those who had been forcibly enfranchised due to previous discriminatory provisions, and to allow bands to control their own band membership as a step towards self-government" (Hanson & Crey, 2009).

Canada, and fight against the Indian Act (Hanson & Crey, 2009).

MODERN DAY

The Canadian public is increasingly aware of Indigenous struggles. This awakening can be exemplified by some recent events. Including the creation of the Truth and Reconciliation committee of Canada that was active between 2008-2015. Their "purpose was [...] documenting the history and lasting impacts of the Canadian residential school system on Indigenous students and their families" (Justice Law Website, n.d, para. 20). In 2019 the National Inquiry into Missing and Murdered Indigenous Women and Girls was published. Revealing that "persistent and deliberate human and Indigenous rights violations and abuses are the root cause behind Canada's staggering rates of violence against Indigenous women, girls and 2SLGBTQQIA people" ("The National Inquiry's Final Report", n.d.). The report called for legal and social changes to resolve the crisis devastating Indigenous communities across Canada. Most recently a series of new unmarked graves across former residential schools containing the remains of Indigenous children from residential schools sparked outrage in Canadians. However, Indigenous peoples in Canada are still fighting (often in court) for equality, their treaty rights, and the rectification of past injustices, with many battles to go.

CONCLUSION

A short chronological journey highlighting key legislative events between British/Canadian – Indigenous relations shows a volatile relationship between Indigenous peoples and what is now Canada. The Royal Proclamation of 1763, and 1764 Treaty of Niagara created relationships between the British Monarchy and Indigenous groups predicated on mutual respect, rights, and territorial integrity. These events set the groundwork for treaty relations, and their subsequent growth. But as time pushed on colonial power grew, war declined, and settlers saw less benefit to their relationship with the Indigenous peoples. Soon colonial powers saw Indigenous peoples as an uncivilised impediment to their objectives. They turned their focus on assimilating Indigenous peoples. With the confederation of Canada came the Indian Act, and its sweeping ability to target status 'Indians' (which includes all beneficiaries of treaties) and enact incredible injustices on them. By 1969 in light of the civil rights movements, Pierre Trudeau consulted Indigenous peoples about their egregious disadvantages, and proposed the White Paper. Largely seen as tone deaf the White Paper seemingly aimed to undo all previous treaties and obligations the government had with Indigenous peoples, and was rejected by Indigenous peoples. Then in 1980 Pierre Trudeau looked to patriate Canada from Britain with a proposed charter that made insufficient mention of Indigenous rights and obligations until these groups advocated for their rights and achieved amendments prior to its codification.

These events illuminate an unjust trajectory for Indigenous peoples in Canada. From a relationship of mutual respect and Wampum belts to residential schools, and the 60's scoop. Indigenous peoples entered treaties in good faith, and were later the subjects of heinous discriminatory practices as a result. Today recognition of these injustices grows, but Indigenous Canadians still fight for rectification of the past, and the upholding of the promises in treaties, of which their promises were fulfilled.

REFERENCES

Crown-Indigenous Relations and Northern Affairs Canada (2016). 250th Anniversary of the Royal Proclamation of 1763. Government of Canada. https://www.rcaanc-cirnac.gc.ca/eng/1370355181092/1607905122267

Crown-Indigenous Relations and Northern Affairs Canada (2020). Treaties and Agreements.Government of Canada. https://www.rcaanc-cirnac.gc.ca/eng/1100100028574/1529354437231

Hanson, E., & Crey, K. (2009). The Indian Act. Indigenous Foundations. https://indigenousfoundations.arts.ubc.ca/the_white_paper_1969/

Hele, K. S. (2021). Treaty of Niagara, 1764. The Canadian Encyclopedia. https://www.thecanadianencyclopedia.ca/en/article/treaty-of-niagara-1764

Justice Law Website (n.d.). The Constitution Acts. Government of Canada. https://laws-lois.justice.gc.ca/eng/const/page-13.html#h-53

Morris, B., & Cassel, J. (2013). the said" Lands…shall be purchased only for Us": The Effect ofthe Royal Proclamation on Government. Active History. https://whttp://activehistory.ca/2013/10/the-said-landsshall-be-purchased-only-for-us-theeffect-of-the-royal-proclamation-on-government/

National Centre for Truth and Reconciliation (n.d.). Residential School History. National Centre for Truth and Reconciliation University of Manitoba. https://nctr.ca/education/teaching-resources/residential-school-history/

Nestor, R. (2018). Pass System in Canada. The Canadian Encyclopedia. https://www.thecanadianencyclopedia.ca/en/article/pass-system-in-canada

Parrott, Z. (2022). Treaties and Agreements. The Canadian Encyclopedia. https://www.thecanadianencyclopedia.ca/en/article/indian-act

Reclaiming Power and Place: The Final Report of the National Inquiry into Missing and Murdered Indigenous Women and Girls. National Inquiry into Missing and Murdered Indigenous Women and Girls. https://www.mmiwg-ffada.ca/final-report/

Statistics Canada (2021). Registered or Treaty Indian Status of Person. Statistics Canada. https://www23.statcan.gc.ca/imdb/p3Var.pl?Function=DEC&Id=42932

CHAPTER 2

ENVIRONMENTAL RACISM AND ITS ASSOCIATED SOCIAL, POLITICAL AND HEALTH CONCERS FOR INDIGENOUS PEOPLE IN CANADA

By Rokya Harun

There continues to be growing concerns regarding various environmental issues present in Canada, which has encouraged an abundance of research and literature on this topic. Moreover, certain groups of individuals and communities are more likely to be exposed to such environmental issues and hazards. Environmental racism occurs when environmental policies and decisions disadvantage racialized individuals, groups, and communities in a disproportionate manner, either intentionally or unintentionally (Venkataraman et al., 2022). Marginalized groups, and Indigenous peoples in particular, are subject to living in environmental conditions that would not be acceptable living conditions for other groups in Canada (Venkataraman et al., 2022). Of the many examples of environmental racism in Canada, there includes the deliberate placement of hazardous waste sites, landfills, incinerators, and polluting industries in lands inhabited by Indigenous communities and other racialized groups (Dhillon & Young, 2010). Consequently, these Indigenous communities are then burdened with illnesses, disease and high incidences of birth defects (Dhillon & Young, 2010). However, research on environmental racism continues to remain scarce compared to the research for general environmental issues (Dhillon & Young, 2010). To combat this, education and awareness of environmental racism must be promoted at the national level, which may increase support for changing the current environmental policies that can be perceived as outdated. Further in-depth research regarding environmental racism affecting Indigenous groups in Canada can bring more insight into the social, political and health impacts. For example, a research paper by Jacobs (2010) explores how racial identities are experienced, internalized and lived with a focus on Indigenous people of Canada. Alongside racism, the exposure to environmental hazards in Canada also intersects with class. Racism affects the lives and experiences of indigenous peoples on their lands, territories, and environment in Canada. For example, environmental racism is evident around First Nations peoples' territories in Canada, such as Fort Chipewyan and Kashechewan (Jacobs, 2010). Reviewing the continuing struggles against the decolonization of Indigenous people in Canada is foundational in understanding environmental racism.

WHAT IS ENVIRONMENTAL RACISM?

Social scientists and environmental activists, including Indigenous Peoples, who were concerned about pollution began to use the term environmental racism in the 1980s in the United States (Jacobs, 2010). Jacobs (2010) continues to explain that race has been a factor in the location of commercial hazardous waste facilities and concluded that patterns of exposure to uncontrolled waste sites for minorities were strong evidence of environmental racism. Environmental racism is an extension of institutional racism (Venkataraman et al., 2022). Institutional racism, also known as systemic racism, is a form of racism that is embedded in the laws and regulations of a society or an organization. Environmental racism involves racial discrimination in environmental policymaking, deliberate targeting of communities of colour for toxic waste and pollutant sites, while excluding these minority groups from the mainstream environmental groups, decision making boards, commissions, and regulatory bodies (Jacobs, 2010). If the consequence of particular regulations puts certain ethnic groups at a disadvantage intendedly or unintendedly, while benefiting the dominant group, then such policies may be designated as systemic forms of discrimination (Jacobs, 2010). Canada, as a government, needs to acknowledge that colonial structures and environmental racism continues to remain in Canada and respond with appropriate and useful legislation that will combat environmental racism (Jacobs, 2010).

INDIGENOUS PEOPLE AND THEIR CONNECTION TO THE LAND AND ENVIRONMENT

Understanding the relationship that indigenous people have to their lands, territories and the environment can further put into perspective the detrimental effects of environmental racism. A significant spiritual, emotional, mental, and physical relationship exists between human beings and their surroundings. Land is not just considered a physical and biological environment by Indigenous people but also an entity consisting of the ashes of their ancestors that must ben conserved for the next seven generations (Jacobs, 2010). Indigenous people have a spiritual connection to "Our Mother the Earth" influencing their belief that humans are no different from plants, animals, trees, and other spiritual things (Jacobs, 2010). A spiritual connection to land is also established through the language of each of the Nations of Indigenous people to communicate who they are in connection with and their relationship with their lands and territories. For instance, in the Ojibwe language, "nishnabe akin" translates to "the land to which the people belong" (Jacobs, 2010). The concept of us belonging to the land is also accompanied by many teachings, such as the mere existence of a relationship between humans and land itself (Jacobs, 2010). Regarding land and environment issues, the Haudenosaunee Clan mothers stated that it is each individual's responsibility to nurture and protect the land (Jacobs, 2010). They continue by stating that the role of being a custodian of the natural world is becoming increasingly challenging for all indigenous people around the world due to growing industrialization destroying Mother Earth (Jacob, 2010). The strong spiritual, physical, mental, and emotional connections maintained by indigenous people arise from their underlying relationship with the land and environment (Jacob, 2010). Indigenous peoples continue to maintain their connections to their surroundings, while resisting the longstanding colonial efforts to deconstruct their practices and beliefs with racist policies embedded within systems.

ENVIRONMENTAL RACISM ROOTED IN COLONIZATION

Indigenous people in Canada suffer from the impacts of both colonization and environmental racism (Jacobs, 2010). They continue to persist with their responsibilities for "Our Mother the Earth", whilst having to adapt to numerous changes in their lands and environment caused by the destruction of their environment intentionally or unintentionally. The enforcement of colonial institutions and laws upon Indigenous peoples marks the beginning of racism in Canada's history. Jacobs (2010) continues to explain how colonization in Canada resulted in the perceived inferiority of Indigenous peoples, which left them with lack of options and control to advocate for themselves whilst having their unjust living conditions ignored or inadequately addressed. The British North America Act from 1867 gave the colonial government unilateral powers to control "Indians" and lands reserved for "Indians" (Jacobs, 2010). This legislation then enabled The Indian Act of 1876 through which the Canadian government imposed a form of institutionalized racism between Canada and its Aboriginal peoples to also allow a form of cultural genocide (Jacobs, 2010). Although Canada is often praised as a progressive and multicultural state, its foundation can be considered to be built upon racist frameworks allowing for the systematic oppression of others by denying or excluding on the basis of race or ethnicity. Jacobs (2010) explains that the Indigenous peoples of the Americas originally intended to share their lands with the European colonial powers, as the land was not theirs to own or to sell. However, Nation-to-nation treaty relationships did acknowledge the Indigenous peoples' relationships to their lands and territories. Despite the treaties, the colonial legal institution did not recognize Indigenous peoples' relationships to their lands (Jacobs, 2010). This "Western vs the Others" complex has enabled Canada to continue with its colonial powers to claim ownership of Indigenous lands and territories to this day. Racist ideologies and legislations have historically made it acceptable to perceive Indigenous peoples as a race that is inherently inferior and incapable of governing themselves. Consequently, traditional lands and ways of life for Indigenous Communities are being compromised on behalf of Canada's economic development through increased logging, mining, dam building, and various other development projects (Jacobs, 2010). Unilateral decisions have been and continue to be solely carried out by the colonial government of Canada without the consent or involvement of Aboriginal peoples, while designating these actions as deemed for their benefit (Jacobs, 2010). As a result, Indigenous communities face barriers when advocating for themselves due to their lack of authority and control over the lands in which they inhabit. The government of Canada must recognize the many instances of Environmental Racism that are ongoing and have impacted the health, social and cultural degradation of Indigenous communities.

EXAMPLES OF ENVIRONMENTAL RACISM AGAINST INDIGENOUS GROUPS

The many examples of environmental racism demonstrated against Indigenous Peoples suggests a need for changes in environmental policies. Dhillon & Young (2010) overviews the many Indigenous communities within Canada that have frequently been victims of environmental racism, such as the Aamjiwnaang, Grassy Narrows, the Kashechewan, and the Pictou Landing First Nation communities. Dhillon & Young (2010) starts by exploring the Aamjiwnaang First Nation in Sarnia, Ontario that are being exposed to larger amounts of toxic air pollutants than average. The Aamjiwnaang reserve, which serves as a host for approximately 850 band members, is deemed as a St. Clair River Area of Concern by the Canada-US Great Lakes International Joint Commission. The Canada's National Pollutant Release Inventory (NPRI) measured that 7.7 million kilograms of Toxic Air Pollutants, that are associated with reproductive, developmental disorders and cancer, were being released in Sarnia in 2005 (Dhillon & Young, 2010). The excessive amounts of pollutants in Sarnia are demonstrated in levels higher than other regions in Ontario and more than the entire provinces of Manitoba, New Brunswick and Saskatchewan combined. Alongside air pollution concerns in Sarnia, the St. Clair River also poses environmental danger despite its water being a source of drinking water for Aamjiwnaang First Nation. The nearly 10 tons of pollutants measured in the St. Clair River was caused as a result of a total of 32 major spills and 300 minor spills occurring between

1974 and 1986. Hundreds of more spills have continued to occur and have been recorded since then. The water quality also worsens due to agricultural runoff and pesticides entering the river. As a consequence of the air and water pollution, increasing evidence demonstrates how the health of Aamjiwnaang First Nation and their local environment have been severely compromised. For example, a survey conducted in 2006 regarding the air pollution in Sarnia found that 40 percent of band members required an inhaler and 17 percent of adults and 22 percent of children reported to have asthma (Dhillon & Young, 2010). The Aamjiwnaang community's cultural life, including hunting, fishing, medicine gathering and ceremonial activities have been affected by the chemical releases. The prolonged years of the community's exposure to air and water pollutants have resulted in a loss of confidence in the support and abilities of their provincial, and federal governments to protect their community from such environmental hazards. Dhillon and Young (2010) proceeds to overview more examples of environmental contamination, which has been a long-standing concern for First Nations people. For example, in 2005, an evacuation of nearly 1000 Kashechewan reserve residents in Ontario was called in response to E.coli bacteria contamination in the reserve's drinking water. A major reason for the E.coli contamination was the installation of the intake pipe for Kashechewan's water treatment plant downstream from a sewage plant. This was accompanied with a lack of on-going maintenance and proper training to prevent repeated contamination of the water supply. 1,900 people on the reserve endured skin infections and chronic illnesses blamed on the poor water quality. To combat the E.coli in the water, the water was treated with excessive amounts of chlorine. However, the chlorine reached "shock" level, which intensified skin irritations leading to burns. This environmental injustice was haphazardly dealt with leading to the relocation of an entire community and also causing further negative social impacts.

There is an overwhelming trend of Indigenous Communities living in environments that have reached beyond the saturation point for exposure to pollutants. For instance, high levels of mercury contamination are found in Indigenous Communities situated near pulp mills, such as the Grass Roots and Pictou Landing First

Nations (Dhillon & Young, 2010). Dhillon & Young (2010) explain that the mercury contamination of the Grassy Narrows was caused by a paper mill in Dryden, Ontario contaminating the English-Wabigoon River system as early as 1970. The Grassy Narrow First Nation community had to endure ongoing health problems due to the consumption of fish contaminated by pulp mill effluent. The mere 9 million dollar compensation by the Government has done little to solve the serious health and social problems faced for over 25 years. Further ignorance has allowed the issue of water contamination to continue with the Pictou Landing First Nation, who had to face the consequences of a nearby pulp mill dumping effluent in their water from 1967 until January 31, 2020 (Lewis et al., 2021). Despite the considerable evidence of environmental degradation faced by Indigenous Communities, many people in Canada and its Government have failed to recognize this as a policy problem requiring urgent attention. The lack of proactivity in dealing with such environmental injustices by failing to recognize, ignoring, or inadequately addressing hazards despite the knowledge of the presence of environmental racism in many indigenous communities has contributed to their decreased quality of life in Canada.

CONSIDERING HEALTH IMPACTS OF ENVIRONMENTAL RACISM

For truth and reconciliation to occur, Canada must also address and remediate the causes and consequences of long term pollution and hazardous sites placed near the land and water of Indigenous communities. A research article by Venkataraman et al. (2022) recognizes the negative physical, emotional, psychological and spiritual health effects that arise due to environmental racism. As a result, health care practitioners (HCPS) must receive appropriate education to address the social, cultural and historical determinants of health by taking into account Canada's historical treatment of Indigenous Peoples. HCPS must have knowledge beyond just the biological health effects of environmental racism and acknowledge where it intersects with other determinants of health, such as low income, housing instability, underemployment and poor access to health care (Venkataraman et al., 2022). Healthcare advocates should be able to identify the determinants of health affecting a community or population, such as recognizing the health care concerns of specific Indigenous communities. For example, when an Indigenous patient presents with cancer or organ damage, this may be related to exposure to toxic chemicals based on where the exposure took place and its effect on the broader community (Venkataraman et al., 2022).

A research study by Lewis et al. (2021) explores how government appointed organizations were undermining the health impacts of pulp mill effluents contaminating the drinking water of the Pictou Landing First Nation (PLFN). Lewis et al. (2021) explains that in 1986, the PLFN filed a lawsuit against the Canadian federal government as they failed their duty to safeguard the interests of the PLFN, who sought compensation for the effluent treatment facility placed on their traditional lands. Alongside an out-of-court settlement reached in 1993 for $35 million, the Pictou Landing Indian Band Agreement Act of 1995 established a Joint Environmental Health Monitoring Committee (JEHMC). The JEHMC is composed of the Department of Indian Affairs, Health Canada, Department of Justice, Environment Canada, and representatives of PLFN (Lewis et al., 2021). Since 1993, the JEHMC has been given the mandate to investigate human and animal health within and near PLFN by examining exposure to toxins in the drinking water, air, and food (Lewis et al., 2021). However, the Indigenous representatives from the community have had little influence in mandating studies that reflect the concerns of their community appropriately. As a result, the Nova Scotia government continued to permit the dumping of pulp mill effluent into a culturally significant body of water bordering PLFN. Lewis et al. (2021) mentions that a human health risk assessment and synthesis report of studies created in relation to the JEHMC concluded there have been no negative impacts on the health of PLFN members from being exposed to 85 million liters of pulp mill effluent dumped per day from 1967 to 2020. Health literature has established that Indigenous health is understood to be inclusive of physical, mental, emotional and spiritual aspects of health, as well as the environment, culture, family, and community. Lewis et al. (2021) developed an environmental health survey that more appropriately assesses the impacts on the PLFN community. They were able to display health impacts through data demonstrating that the four dimensions of health are not in balance for the PLFN when employing a survey that considered a more culturally appropriate definition of health. For example, one-half (50%) of all PLFN participants report that they have felt down or depressed in the past year. However, Lewis et al. (2021) recognized that the self-reported feelings of depression are higher than expected since mental health issues typically impact one in five people (20%) of the population. Lewis et al. (2021) also found that impacts of racism are significant across all dimensions of health. For example, those who have not experienced racism are healthier (84%) than those who have experienced it (56%).

Institutional racism, enabled by colonialism, continues to shape environmental policies and practices today (Venkataraman et al., 2022). For instance, numerous Indigenous communities in Canada continue to have long-term advisories implemented regarding their drinking water (Venkataraman et al., 2022). Although it is the federal government's responsibility to address the lack of access to clean drinking water for many Indigenous communities, they have fallen short thus far to create proper and realistic solutions (Venkataraman et al., 2022). As a result, further revision of environmental policies and frameworks are required to address the environmental injustices faced by Indigenous communities.

NEED FOR REVISING POLICIES TO ADDRESS ENVIRONMENTAL RACISM IN INDIGENOUS COMMUNITIES

To ensure effective policy changes, Indigenous peoples who are most affected by these policies must be included in discussions of environmental policy changes. This will allow for policies to take into account Indigenous teachings and ways of life that focus on whole person care, our connections to land, protecting life and maintaining harmony with nature (Venkataraman et al., 2022). An example of an attempt for policy change includes Bill C-230 (Venkataraman et al., 2022). Bill C-230 was a federal bill that sought to require the Ministry of the Environment, government representatives, and Indigenous and other affected communities to create a strategy to redress environmental racism. This bill would be used to identify and prioritize the cleanup of contaminated sites in areas where Indigenous Peoples, racialized and low-income Canadians live (Venkataraman et al., 2022). However, the bill did not become law and died with the dissolution of the Parliament in 2021 (Venkataraman et al., 2022). For general policy changes, there needs to be a focus on reducing cases of environmental injustice, promoting awareness of environmental protection methods, and/or increasing responsibilities of current regulatory bodies overseeing environmental assessments to also include regulation of environmental justice issues, such as environmental racism (Dhillon & Young, 2010).

People across Canada can help garner support for sustainable changes by educating themselves on Canada's colonial history and recognizing the existence of past and ongoing environmental racism occurring against Indigenous communities (Venkataraman et al., 2022). Moving forward, Canada must learn from their mistakes and be able to address the health of Indigenous communities from a proactive and preventive standpoint rather than responding reactively to the consequences of Indigenous communities suffering from prolonged exposure to excess environmental hazards being placed within and near their lands.

REFERENCES

Dhillon, C., & Young, M. G. (2010). Environmental racism and First Nations: A call for socially just public policy development. Canadian Journal of Humanities and Social Sciences, 1(1), 25-39. https://www.researchgate.net/profile/Michael-Young-46/publication/228226535_Environmental_Racism_and_First_Nations_A_Call_for_Socially_Just_Public_Policy_Development/links/568aa6f808ae1e63f1fbe044/Environmental-Racism-and-First-Nations-A-Call-for-Socially-Just-Public-Policy-Development.pdf

Jacobs, B. (2010, May). Environmental racism on Indigenous lands and territories. In Canadian Political Science Association Annual Conference (Vol. 29).https://www.cpsa-acsp.ca/papers-2010/Jacobs.pdf

Lewis, D., Francis, S., Francis-Strickland, K., Castleden, H., & Apostle, R. (2021). If only they had accessed the data: Governmental failure to monitor pulp mill impacts on human health in Pictou Landing First Nation. Social Science & Medicine, 288, 113184.https://doi.org/10.1016/j.socscimed.2020.113184

Venkataraman, M., Grzybowski, S., Sanderson, D., Fischer, J., & Cherian, A. (2022).Environmental racism in Canada. Canadian Family Physician, 68(8), 567. https://www.cfp.ca/content/cfp/68/8/567.full.pdf

CHAPTER 3

ISSUES IN ACCESS TO AND PROVISION OF HEALTHCARE FOR INDIGENOUS PEOPLE IN CANADA

By Maria Ashraf

"Of all the forms of inequality, injustice in health care is the most shocking and inhumane." -Dr. Martin Luther King

INTRODUCTION

Having good health is one of the most necessary steps to leading a fulfilled life. However, the maintenance of health is not as simple as it sounds. While being such an integral part of life and an essential human right, the idea of having good health is still alien to many. The reasons behind this are many. On one hand, there is a severe disparity in healthcare provision and access. On the other hand, the concept of mainstream healthcare and health may not be interchangeable around different cultures and communities. These two issues and many others have detrimental consequences for human life throughout various communities around the world. Furthermore, the impact of these issues can be very specific to each community and its situation. Thus, to dissect the issue of inequity in healthcare provision and access it is essential to be mindful of the specificity and history of each community or individual being discussed. This chapter will focus on the issue of healthcare access and provision faced by indigenous people and communities in Canada (the following chapter will discuss mental health issues in more detail). It will begin with a discussion on the importance of healthcare and health. Then it will move on to describe healthcare across indigenous communities in Canada and the current issues they face. To conclude, the chapter will end with suggestions for solutions and a discussion on future directions.

THE MEANING OF HEALTH AND HEALTHCARE

Health today can have multiple definitions, it may just mean the absence of disease or it may also mean living in complete harmony with one's environment (Sartorius, 2006). The definition of health this chapter will revolve around is the World Health Organization's (WHO) understanding of Health. The WHO describes health as "Health is a state of complete physical, mental and social well-being and not merely the absence of disease or infirmity" (World Health Organization, n.d.). This definition broadens how health is viewed. Having good health does not merely mean that one is free from an illness or disease, it also encompasses the concept of being able to enjoy a holistic state of harmony and wellbeing in all life aspects. Consequently, this view of health also modifies the perspective through which one may view healthcare and its access. Going by the traditional definition of health and the absence of disease, access to healthcare may symbolise a simple solution to eliminating health issues. However, the broad definition of health views this concept with far more complexity. It views health with a holistic lens and thus healthcare, its access, and its provision must be compatible and holistic as well.

IMPORTANCE OF HEALTH AND HEALTHCARE FOR COMMUNITIES

To begin, as aforementioned good health is such a vital aspect of leading a good life. Health is an aspect of life that is interconnected with and interwoven into almost all parts of life. From physiological well-being dictating the quality of life to mental well-being relating to emotions and thinking, good health is at the core of living a fulfilled life. Health is also at the core of major human life milestones. Good health is necessary for achieving a higher quality of life, for achieving better life expectancy and being able to experience life with efficiency and

BARRIERS TO THE ACHIEVEMENT OF GOOD HEALTH

So, how does one achieve good health? Is there a way to achieve good health solely as an individual? Well, the unfortunate answer is no. The main rationale behind this is due to, again, the nature of health. Health today is dependent on so many aspects that are beyond individual control. These aspects do not only include environmental factors, but social and economic factors also play a role. Specifically, these factors are also known as socioeconomic determinants of health. The World Health Organization refers to these as "the conditions in which people are born, grow, live, work and age" (Braveman & Gottlieb, 2014). Some examples of these factors include ethnicity, income, social status, education, employment status and conditions, housing, food security, etc. All of these factors go beyond the personal responsibility of an individual in achieving good health status. With such diversity and complexity, the attainment of good health in part is heavily dependent on regular access to healthcare. However, regular access to healthcare is not available for many due to variances in how healthcare is provided and made available to communities across the world. While ideally, healthcare access is a universal human right, its distribution, unfortunately, depends on factors beyond basic humanity. Healthcare today depends on several social, economic, and political factors. With this inequity, healthcare access is an issue that leaves many underresourced communities vulnerable to health issues and without concrete solutions.

INDIGENOUS COMMUNITIES AND HEALTHCARE ISSUES

The issue of healthcare access and provision in indigenous communities in Canada has been major and growing. The status of public health policies and healthcare in Canada for Indigenous people can be reflected by the fact that the Canadian Public Health Association considers aboriginal status a determinant of health (Canadian Public Health Association, n.d.). That is if one merely belongs to an indigenous community, one's health and healthcare will be significantly impacted by it. Furthermore, studies carried out by statistics Canada highlighted additional issues with healthcare and access in indigenous populations. Firstly, indigenous populations have a higher incidence rate of chronic health issues (Hahmann & Kumar, 2022) . Additionally, Hahmann, Badets, & Hughes, found in 2019 that indigenous populations in Canada suffer from more disability and disability-related illnesses compared to other populations. In addition to more chronic illness and health issues, indigenous health has been greatly impacted by socioeconomic factors of income, substance abuse, colonial abuse, poverty, and social injustice (Hayward et. al, 2020). In addition to merely causing mental and physical health problems, these issues also add to chronic disease and even lead to more issues that may not have been present without the social and colonial history of indigenous populations. Furthermore, another issue indigenous populations face in terms of healthcare is gender disparity in the prevalence of the disease. For example, certain illnesses are more prevalent in indigenous women such as arthritis, mental health issues, asthma, etc. Similarly, women also report weakened immune systems (Hahmann & Kumar, 2022). All of these issues can again be traced back to social factors such as racism, colonialism, and racism (Hahmann & Kumar, 2022). Thus, the issue of indigenous is very complex and to address the issues in healthcare it is essential to introduce the issues in health. The main issues this chapter will focus on are access and provision.

ISSUES WITH ACCESS

The issue with access to healthcare in indigenous communities is complex and multifaceted. Before going into details of the issues with access it is important to promptly describe what healthcare access means. Healthcare access can mean simply having health services available, however, that does not translate into having adequate access to healthcare. The reason is that even if there is an adequate supply of health services, the proper and advantageous use is dependent on additional factors such as relevancy to the community, physical access, affordability, and acceptability of services by the community (Gulliford et al., 2002). While these additional factors impact issues of access to healthcare beyond merely the supply of services, one of the major issues faced by indigenous communities are the lack of available health services.

GEOGRAPHICAL ISSUES

The first major issue indigenous peoples face is the geographical barrier to accessing health services. Access to health services is strongly reliant on one's physical location and proximity to health services. In terms of most of the indigenous population in Canada and their distribution, it is very difficult for most indigenous people to access good health facilities close to them. While most indigenious populations are distributed across urban areas a major part of the population resides in remote and underresourced areas. For example, around one-third of all indigenous peoples in Canada (First Nations people, Métis and Inuit) reside in rural areas. Additionally, at least 19% reside in smaller communities. This geographical distribution of the population impacts healthcare access for at least one-third of indigenous populations. Rural areas in Canada currently face many issues in providing supply and matching the adequate demand for healthcare. For example, one of the major issues faced by rural areas in Canada is the availability of physicians. In terms of statistics, in a paper published by Can Fam Physician, it was highlighted that only 8% of Canada's total doctors serve rural areas (Wilson et. al., 2020). This highlights that one of the major flaws in healthcare access is the lack of a primary factor, having access to physicians. This lack does not only mean that patients do not have access to medical professionals when an issue arises but also highlights the absence of regular care and checkups.

Regular check-ups are necessary for the promotion of health and the efficiency of health services. Even if there are hospitals and clinics, if there are no physicians available for the care of patients there are issues with health access. In addition to this being a geographical issue, this issue is prevalent in indigenous populations. For example, it was found in a study about diabetes done by Shah et. al. in 2020, that First Nations people had lower rates of having access to a regular family physician compared to other populations in Ontario. The rate of indigenous patients was 85.3% vs 97.7%. Furthermore, indigenous peoples also scored lower in terms of continuity of care with a family physician and were less likely to see and have access to specialists. Furthermore, geography and isolation also lead to other issues in accessing alternative forms of healthcare. Some rural areas do not have access to high-speed internet and communication services which makes it difficult to provide alternative forms of medicine such as virtual care. Lastly, geographic isolation also equates to delays in receiving immediate help without considerable travel. This is very dangerous, especially when it comes to emergencies such as accidents, heart attacks, strokes, etc. that require immediate advanced health care.

SYSTEMIC BARRIERS

In addition to actual physical barriers when it comes to healthcare access a significant amount of hurdles come from systematic barriers that indigenous people face in the Canadian healthcare system. While the Canadian healthcare system is labelled as a universal healthcare system access to its services is not uniform for all. The way Indigenous peoples are prevented from receiving equal access may not be a deliberate practice and is rather a failure of the health system and its policies. These policies, systems, and methods are not deliberately set up to prevent access but are not inclusive of the distinctive health and social issues of indigenous people.

COLONIALISM AND ITS IMPACT

Before diving into the specific systemic barriers faced by indigenous people. It is necessary to establish the root causes behind them. One of the most profound and widely discussed causes of systemic barriers and their prevalence is colonialism. Colonialism can be defined as "a policy or set of policies and practices where a political power from one territory exerts control in a different territory. It involves unequal power relations." (FemNorthNet, 2016). Indigenous people faced colonialism when European settlers began taking away their lands, culture, and societies and began to replace them with their own. This sad history was not just European settlers establishing a new country and working towards economic development but this also led to the subtle eradication of indigenous people's land, power, and culture. Historical trauma from colonisation like this is bound to have impacts in the present and future. Not only did this colonisation itself change the position of indigenous people in the fabric of society but it also developed a deep divide in their relationship with this new society. Thus, not only does colonisation attempt to erase and destruct indigenous culture and identity but it also begins to control society and make indigenous people dependent on their own culture, ideas, and practices (Nguyen et.al., 2020).

So how does this impact healthcare access? Well, healthcare in itself is a social phenomenon, especially in the context of Canadian Society. In Canada, accessing and utilising healthcare is a social task at all levels. It is a relationship between an individual, the government, and society. Colonisation has not only destroyed this relationship but has also made it incredibly difficult to establish. This eventually leads to the establishment and intensification of systemic barriers.

SYSTEMIC RACISM

One of the most prevalent and serious systemic barriers to accessing healthcare is systemic racism. What is systemic racism? The University of British Columbia (UBC) describes systemic racism in Canada as "In a settler colonial state like Canada, systemic racism is deeply rooted in every system of this country. This means the systems put in place were designed to benefit white colonists while disadvantaged the Indigenous populations who had lived here prior to colonialism. This power dynamic continues to be upheld and reinforced in our society, extending its impact on new racialized citizens." (UBC, n.d.). This statement clearly describes what systemic racism looks like in Canada and what it looks like for indigenous patients. Another concrete example of this is an article by the Canadian Broadcasting Corporation (CBC) that highlighted an allegation that healthcare providers in an emergency room would play a 'guessing game' in which they would try to guess the blood alcohol level of incoming indigenous patients (Schmunk , 2020). Furthermore, the article also shares conclusions from a study done on indigenous people that highlighted the impact of racism in healthcare. The study named 'First Peoples, Second Class Treatment' was done in 2015 (Schmunk , 2020). According to its findings, because Indigenous people encounter such a high level of racism from medical professionals, they frequently plan to deal with it before going to emergency rooms or steer clear of hospitals completely (Schmunk , 2020). Examples like this highlight how systemic racism leads to issues in proper healthcare access in various ways. Firstly, it takes away the trust a patient needs to have in the healthcare system. If indigenous peoples face so much racism that a hospital visit would stress them out or they would even consider not going, it means that the healthcare system is not accessible to them. If a system in place is something that would rather not be used because of its flawed design or the detrimental impacts that come with its use then such a system is a failed system. In addition, systemic racism goes beyond making the actual system unnavigable for indigenous people. The system itself is rooted in racist policies and notions. When racism exists in a system, it does not only impact one policy it seeps into every action, every idea, and every person. If the very healthcare providers that are supposed to care for and build trust with their patients hold discriminatory views, then the patients do not have access to a fair and equitable system.

ISSUES WITH HEALTHCARE PROVISION

Adding to the previous discussion, it is important to note that healthcare access is deeply tied to issues with healthcare provision. While healthcare access is more focused on how healthcare services are made available, provision is focused on actually providing those services. This section of the chapter will focus on some issues regarding providing equitable healthcare.

LACK OF INCLUSIVE PROFESSIONAL HEALTHCARE EDUCATION

One of the biggest issues with providing proper healthcare to indigenous individuals lies in the fact that Canada's healthcare providers are not educated with an inclusive curriculum that focuses on the issues of indigenous people and navigating the healthcare issues they face. While there have been many recommendations for changing curriculums for healthcare providers, the actual progress and teaching of the curriculum are still in the works (Blanchet et al., 2021). The reason this is so essential is to create more empathetic healthcare professionals that can provide inclusive care to indigenous patients. Thus, Beyond simply increasing public awareness of the poor treatment of Indigenous patients by the healthcare system, it is crucial to work toward understanding the broader racism ingrained in societal norms, organisational cultures, and legal frameworks (Blanchet et al., 2021).

LACK OF INCLUSIVE POLICIES

With such a complex and substantial history of colonization and discrimination, it is imminent that the healthcare needs of indigenous people are an exception to the rest of society and require more consideration. The current healthcare system is thus incompatible with catering to the needs of indigenous people. An additional reason why inclusive healthcare provision is challenging is the lack of inclusive policies. As aforementioned, indigenous people's history and relationship with the healthcare system are unique and require special consideration. Currently, there is no specific legislation or policy that focuses on improving indigenous health in Canada (Gouldhawke, 2022). In the past, the 2004 Health Accord was a 10-year plan focused on improving indigenous healthcare experiences (Gouldhawke, 2022). However, that plan has long expired in 2014 and has yet to find its replacement. This significant lack of a targeted policy is one of the major reasons why indigenous healthcare provision has been challenging (Gouldhawke, 2022). The reason a policy is important is that it shapes the way decisions are taken, funding is allocated, and action is taken. In short, it highlights whether an issue will get significance on a larger scale or not. Thus, the lack of inclusive policies is also a hurdle in providing healthcare to indigenous populations.

SUGGESTIONS AND FUTURE TRENDS

As highlighted throughout the chapter, the healthcare needs of indigenous populations in Canada are not a simple issue. This issue is rooted in colonial history, racism, and a lack of awareness of indigenous issues and identities. The solution to these problems thus involves more than just band-aid solutions. There is a lack of action when it comes to indigenous issues. As previously mentioned, even when there are suggestions for making the healthcare system more inclusive, follow-up actions are lacking. Some possible modifications will be discussed next.

SOLUTIONS TO GEOGRAPHICAL BARRIERS

In order to improve the access to healthcare for indigenous communities it is necessary to work on integrating them with communities. The Canadian government should work on issues such as investing in transportation and road infrastructure (Nguyen et. al., 2020). Additionally, they should focus on building more hospitals and accessible healthcare centres in remote communities.

SOLUTIONS TO SYSTEMIC BARRIERS

In order to solve the issue of systemic barriers, it is necessary to educate and reform the entire healthcare system and society as a whole. With such a broad goal, this solution will require multiple multifaceted approaches and solutions. However, the most important is to fix the issues of systemic racism and understand the impact of colonialism on indigenous populations.

SOLUTIONS FOR HEALTHCARE PROVISION

The main solution for better healthcare provision is to train and create better healthcare providers through increased efforts in provider education and policy. The biggest gaps in provision stem from an overall lack of awareness and absence of action.

CONCLUSION

In essence, healthcare access and provision in indigenous communities is an integral topic. Focusing on this topic is essential because it helps answer questions like, why do indigenous people have lower survival rates? Why do they have a high prevalence of chronic illness? Why are they avoiding doctors? How are doctors treating them? And lastly, what can we do about it? This topic is a crucial topic for the betterment of not only indigenous communities but also the greater Canadian society. It is time that Canadian society acknowledges the inequity present in the treatment of indigenous people and takes strong and sustainable corrective action towards it.

REFERENCES

Blanchet Garneau, A., Bélisle, M., Lavoie, P., & Laurent Sédillot, C. (2021). Integrating equity and social justice for indigenous peoples in undergraduate health professions education in Canada: a framework from a critical review of literature. International journal for equity in health, 20(1), 123. https://doi.org/10.1186/s12939-021-01475-6

Braveman, P., & Gottlieb, L. (2014). The social determinants of health: it's time to consider the causes of the causes. Public health reports (Washington, D.C. : 1974), 129 Suppl 2(Suppl 2), 19–31. https://doi.org/10.1177/00333549141291S206

Canadian Public Health Association. (n.d.). What are the social determinants of health? Canadian Public Health Association | Association Canadienne de Santé Publique. Retrieved November 12, 2022, from https://www.cpha.ca/what-are-social-determinants-health

FemNorthNet. (2016). Colonialism and its Impacts. Resource Development in Northern Communities: Local Women Matter #3. Ottawa: Canadian Research Institute for the Advancement of Women

Gouldhawke, M. (2022, May 30). The failure of Federal Indigenous Healthcare Policy in Canada. Yellowhead Institute. Retrieved December 2, 2022, from https://yellowheadinstitute.org/2021/02/04/the-failure-of-federal-indigenous-healthcare-p olicy-in-canada/

Gulliford, M., Figueroa-Munoz, J., Morgan, M., Hughes, D., Gibson, B., Beech, R., & Hudson, M. (2002). What does 'access to health care' mean?. Journal of health services research & policy, 7(3), 186–188. https://doi.org/10.1258/135581902760082517 Sartorius N. (2006). The meanings of health and its promotion. Croatian medical journal, 47(4), 662–664.

Hayward, Cidro, Dutton, & Passey, 2020, https://www150.statcan.gc.ca/n1/pub/89-653-x/89-653-x2019005-eng htm

Hahmann & Kumar, 2022. Unmet health care needs during the pandemic and resulting impacts among First Nations people living off reserve, Métis and Inuit https://www150.statcan.gc.ca/n1/pub/45-28-0001/2022001/article/00008-eng.htm

Nguyen, N. H., Subhan, F. B., Williams, K., & Chan, C. B. (2020). Barriers and Mitigating Strategies to Healthcare Access in Indigenous Communities of Canada: A Narrative Review. Healthcare (Basel, Switzerland), 8(2), 112. https://doi.org/10.3390/healthcare8020112

Schmunk , R. (2020, June 20). B.C. investigating allegations ER staff played 'game' to guess blood-alcohol level of indigenous patients | CBC News. CBCnews. Retrieved December 3, 2022, from https://www.cbc.ca/news/canada/british-columbia/racism-in-bc-healthcare-health-ministe r-adrian-dix-1.5619245

Shah, B. R., Slater, M., Frymire, E., Jacklin, K., Sutherland, R., Khan, S., Walker, J. D., & Green, M. E. (2020). Use of the health care system by Ontario First Nations people with diabetes: a population-based study. CMAJ open, 8(2), E313–E318. https://doi.org/10.9778/cmajo.20200043

UBC. (n.d.). Systemic racism: What it looks like in Canada and how to fight it?. Vice-President Finance & Operations Portfolio (VPFO). Retrieved December 3, 2022, from https://vpfo.ubc.ca/2021/03/systemic-racism-what-it-looks-like-in-canada-and-how-to-fight-it/

Wilson, C. R., Rourke, J., Oandasan, I. F., Bosco, C., On behalf of the Rural Road Map Implementation Committee, & Au nom du Comité sur la mise en œuvre du Plan d'action sur la médecine rurale (2020). Progress made on access to rural health care in Canada [Progrès réalisés dans l'accès aux soins de santé ruraux au Canada]. Canadian Family Physician, 66(1), 31–36.

World Health Organization. (n.d.). Constitution of the World Health Organization. World Health Organization. Retrieved November 5, 2022, from https://www.who.int/about/governance/constitution

CHAPTER 4

MENTAL HEALTH AND ITS ASSOCIATED CONCERNS IN INDIGENOUS PEOPLE

By Hafsa Binte Younus

INTRODUCTION

This chapter talks about mental health concerns in the Indeginous people. It talks about the factors that lead to mental health concern in these communities. It also discusses the common mental health concerns and some of the barriers faced by these communities.

The term "indigenous people" refers to three groups that are recognized by the Constitution act which include First Nation people, Metis, and Inuits. They along with their communities, cultures, and languages have existed way before the land that we reside on today was even known as Canada. However, the people of these communities have experienced rapid cultural changes, marginalisation, and absorption into the global community with little regard for their autonomy. This cultural discontinuity has been linked to high rates of mental health issues in these communities. This chapter will explore the mental health issues of the indigenous people of Canada (Graham et al., 2021).

WHAT IS MENTAL HEALTH

According to the World Health Organization, "Mental health is a state of mental well-being that enables people to cope with the stresses of life, realise their abilities, learn well and work well, and contribute to their community" (WHO, 2022). It refers to the cognitive, behavioural, emotional, and social well-being of an individual. It is about how a person thinks, feels, and behaves (CDC, 2021). It helps determine how an individual deals with stress, relates with others and makes healthy decisions (CDC, 2021). It impacts an individual's life by affecting their daily living, physical and emotional health, as well as their relationships with others (CDC, 2021). Just like physical health, mental health is just as important. This is because both physical and mental health has an impact on each other and having poor mental health can lead to an increased risk of physical health problems.

There are many risk factors that may lead to developing a poor mental health or mental health disorders. Some of these include early adverse life experiences such as a history of abuse or trauma (i.e. child abuse, sexual assault, witnessing violence), biological factors such as genetics and chemical imbalances in the brain, the use of drugs and alcohol, experiences related to ongoing medical conditions such as cancer and diabetes, family history, as well as social and financial circumstances such as poverty, violence, inequality and environmental deprivation (Tee-Melegrito et al., 2022). Risks can manifest themselves at all stages of life but those occurring during these sensitive developmental periods, especially during early childhood are particularly detrimental to an individual's mental health. Some signs of having good mental health include the following: taking pride in who you are, enjoying life, being able to form as well as manage satisfying relationships, being able to cope with problems and stress in a positive way, always driving to realise your potential, and having a sense of personal control (Government of Canada; Indigenous Services Canada, 2022).

MENTAL HEALTH IN INDIGENOUS PEOPLE

Today, the indigenous people constitute about 1.8 million people which make up around 5% of the total population in Canada (Government of Canada, 2022). However, suffering from violence, racism, inequality, ignorance, stereotypes, and historical government interventions, the indigenous people in Canada deal with serious mental health challenges. Although the health and well-being of indigenous people in Canada have improved significantly over the past few years, these communities continue to have higher rates of poor Mental Health, suicide, infant mortality, diabetes, obesity, food insecurity, and lower life expectancy (Kirmayer et al., 2000). As compared to the non-indigenous population, the Indigenous population is twice as likely to experience Mental Health issues. They overall have poorer mental health outcomes including anxiety, depression, and suicide (Kirmayer et al., 2000).

Although the indigenous people in general have poorer Mental Health outcomes, the outcomes of mental health amongst First Nations, Inuits, and the Metis people have been found to be different. For example, according to CAMH, especially the youth of indigenous people die by suicide at a much higher rate than non-indigenous people. First Nation youth ages 15 to 24 die by suicide about 6 times more than non-indigenous youth. Moreover, the rate of suicide among the Inuit youth is about 24 times more than the national average rate of suicides. Geographical location also seems to play a role in determining the mental health of a particular community. For example, first Nation people living on reserves were found to have suicide rates twice that of those living off reserves. Approximately 1 in 4 First Nation youth and one in five First Nation adults living on reserves report psychological distress linked to moderate to severe mental health disorders (*Mental illness and addiction: Facts and statistics*, n.d.).

One of the major factors that have severely negatively impacted the mental health of indigenous people is the historical, systematic, and systemic colonialism instituted in Canada which was done to assimilate all indigenous people (Morton Ninomiya et al., 2020). This has caused severe intergenerational harms that have been having ongoing and long-term negative effects on the health of indigenous people which has been passed down from one generation to the next generation (Morton Ninomiya et al., 2020). The indigenous people have been severely affected by the loss of their land, culture, and language as well as forced assimilation, violence, marginalisation, racist policies, and chronic trauma. Studies have shown that cultural discontinuity has been linked to higher rates of depression alcoholism suicide and violence in many communities, especially in the use of the communities (Morton Ninomiya et al., 2020). They also experience ongoing stressors including large social economic disparities, discrimination, racism, oppression, and inequalities. All this has resulted in them experiencing grief and other emotional distresses leading to mental health issues (Morton Ninomiya et al., 2020).

A British Columbia Aboriginal survivor study examined the abuse mental health and health profiles of 127 Aboriginal survivors of residential school systems (Corrado & Cohen, 2003). The main age of the subjects when they arrived at the residential school was around 8.5 years and were around 15 years of age when they left the residential school. Many of the students belonged to intact families before coming to residential schools however only a small minority of them return to intact families (Corrado & Cohen, 2003). Residential institutions were described as total institutions where a large number of Aboriginal children lived and worked together while being separated from their societies and the broader Canadian society as a whole (Corrado & Cohen, 2003). The schools were intended to undermine the culture of those Aboriginal children in order to "civilise" them (Corrado & Cohen, 2003). They were stripped of all their belongings including artifacts of their culture, clothes as well as hairstyles as soon as they arrived at the residential schools (Corrado & Cohen, 2003). They were forbidden to speak their native language or practice their cultural traditions and were punished in the form of corporal punishments which included whipping. They were forced to leave their cultural background behind by being forced to practice Christianity, learn basic mathematics, farm, and use the English language (Corrado & Cohen, 2003). Four major categories of abuse were identified in the literature involving residential schools which included physical sexual psychological and spiritual abuse. The study found that of the 127 residential school survivors who were examined only two of them were free of mental illness (Corrado & Cohen, 2003). Almost 30.4% of the survivors experienced major depressive episodes, 26.1% of them experienced chronic depression, and over 64.2% of the survivors experienced post-traumatic stress disorder (Corrado & Cohen, 2003).

There are only a few rigorous studies on the mental health of Canadian native indigenous people. The flower of two soil project was one of the best studies which examined the relationship between academic performance psychosocial variables and mental health and Aboriginal children. It also compared it with mental health factors affecting non-native control children at several sites across the United States and Canada. This study examined the symptoms of depression and conduct disorder in children. It was found that by both parents and teachers native children especially the boys were more often to be classified as having symptoms of conduct disorder as compared to non-native children (MacMillan et al., 1996).

In 1997 the First Nation and Inuit Regional Health service was conducted across Canada (excluding Alberta and the northern and James Bay region of Quebec). The survey included questions addressing mental health and well-being but it lacked diagnostic measures which made it impossible to estimate the rate of psychiatric disorders. From the survey, it was found that almost 17% of parents reported that the child of their community had emotional or behavioural problems as compared to other children from non-indigenous communities (Kirmayer et al., 2000).

MOST COMMON MENTAL HEALTH CONCERNS IN THE INDIGENOUS POPULATION

One of the most dramatic indicators of distress in the Aboriginal population is suicide. As described above, the Aboriginal communities have elevated suicide rates, particularly among youth. The reason behind the elevated suicide rate includes biological psychological and social factors. Although they are very individual factors that may play a role in the poor mental health of many youths, social factors such as inequality and stereotype as well as historical factors and events such as the residential school event also play a role as young generations also experience the effect of the historical trauma. These individuals who went to residential schools lost their sense of identity, culture, and language (*Residential schools*, 2022). The communities experienced a great amount of trauma as parents who were forced to send their children to residential schools had to deal with the devastating effect of separation from the children and the lack of input in the care and welfare of the children. They also had to deal with the constant fear and worry about the safety of their children. Many of the children suffered emotional physical and sexual abuse from staff and were forced to let go of their language and culture. This in addition led to the feelings of alienation, anger, and shame which were passed down to the next generations. The impact of the trauma that came with the residential school experience was intergenerational and passed on from one generation to the next generation (*Residential schools,* 2022). Studies have shown that children of parents who attended the Indian residential school (IRS) had an increased risk of suicidal thoughts and attempts in adolescence and adulthood (Bombay et al., 2018). The study showed that females were negatively affected by the parents who attended the Indian residential school however male children of those parents had a greater link with suicide Ideation (Bombay et al., 2018). The second survey of the study showed that female youth who had parents who attend Indian Residential Schools had a significantly greater relation with social ideation (Bombay et al., 2018). The influence of parental attendance in Indian residential schools was strong amongst youth aged 12 to 14 as compared to those aged 15 to 17 years old (Bombay et al., 2018). The impact of Intergeneral trauma was reinforced by the racist attitudes that continue to permeate Canadian societies (Bombay et al., 2018).

Another common mental health issue in the Indigenous community is depression. Depression is a mood disorder that causes persistent feelings of sadness and loss of interest which interferes with an individual's ability to do normal day-to-day activities. It may also lead to a person feeling worthless. It can be a result of upsetting life events, being sick, or having changes to personal life or environment. Studies have shown that compared to non-indigenous communities, the depression rates amongst the indigenous community are much higher for both males and females residing either on or off reserve. The colonisation-enforced assimilation of indigenous people in Canada is considered to be the cause of depression in these communities too. For example removal of children from their families over consecutive generations resulted in broken attachment relationships which is a significant factor in the development of depression in many Aboriginal people in

Canada. Many studies show that childhood separation from parents is associated with an increased risk of depression in adulthood. This broken parent-child attachment style can be linked to depression as it impacts both the child's biological system that is responsible for resilience to stress as well as the development of their view of self in relation to others (Bellamy & Hardy, 2015).

Indigenous communities also had a higher risk of substance use disorder due to a variety of reasons including historical and structural Injustice. According to the Canadian census mortality follow-up study, tobacco smoking-related causes was significantly higher than the Metis population as compared to the non-indigenous population with it being 75% higher amongst Metis females and 14% higher amongst Metis males. A study compared the pattern of tobacco, alcohol, and marijuana use among indigenous youth attending off-reserve schools to non indigenous youth. It was found that indigenous youth were more significantly likely to be current smokers as compared to non-indigenous youth. Moreover, indigenous youth smokers were also more likely than non-indigenous youth to have ever tried to quit smoking. In terms of alcohol use, indigenous youth were reported to start drinking at a slightly younger age than non-indigenous students. The same results were found for marijuana use with non-indigenous students being less likely to have ever tried marijuana as compared to indigenous students. The study also concluded that although the rates of smoking alcohol and marijuana had decreased in both the indigenous and the non-indigenous populations, the gap between the two populations was not with indigenous youth having higher odds of abusing substances as compared to non-indigenous youth. There could be many factors that could have been an influence such as past intergenerational trauma, lack of resources and opportunities, lack of proper programs in place, and so on (Sikorski et al., 2019).

MENTAL HEALTH SINCE THE BEGINNING OF COVID

According to Statistics Canada, the covid-19 pandemic has resulted in huge social disruptions which have led many to struggle with changes to routine and feelings of uncertainty. Findings have shown the negative impacts of the covid-19 pandemic on the mental health of the indigenous participants too. 6 and 10 indigenous participants reported that their mental health had worsened since the beginning of social distancing. Amongst the crowdsource indigenous participants 38% reported fair or poor mental health 32 reported good mental health and 31 reported excellent or very good mental health. However, when asked how their mental health has changed since the beginning of social distancing 60% of the indigenous participants reported that their mental health had become somewhat worse or much worse. Especially indigenous women especially reported higher levels of stress and anxiety. As compared to people of non-indigenous communities the crowdsource that reflected mental health concerns were reported to be higher in the indigenous population. 40% of indigenous participants describe most days as being quite stressful or extremely stressful and 41% reported symptoms consistent with moderate or high anxiety as compared to 27 and 25% of non-indigenous participants. This disparity in the mental health effect of covid-19 could be linked to intergeneration effects of residential schools, Force relocation, mental health service gaps, and other stressors such as childhood adversity, trauma, and discrimination (Arriagada et al., 2020).

BARRIERS TO MENTAL HEALTH CARE

Formal services are often alighted and informal supports are often used as the first choice for seeking help. Studies have shown that participants report being more comfortable talking to family and friends as compared to psychologists or counsellors. In a study of 74 American Indian service consumers, a quarter of the meal participants were willing to talk about their problems with their family or friends; however, less than 10 persons were willing to talk about their problems with the doctors. In terms of females, more than 1/3 were willing to talk to their family about their problems, however less than 10% were willing to talk to a doctor or a counsellor. This shows that one of the biggest barriers to getting professional Mental Health services is the lack of willingness of the participants themselves to go to a professional counsellor as they prefer talking to a family or a friend. Although many participants prefer talking to a family or a friend, they still had a positive attitude toward getting professional help if things were perceived as serious (Goetz et al., 2022).

Another barrier includes structural obstacles and support. In availability of needed Mental Health services and resources for indigenous clients have been one of the major concerns. Not having access to indigenous service providers along with language barriers as well as long wait lists are factors that further contribute to barriers. Moreover, lack of resources such as having fewer computers also leads to further adding to this barrier as this leads to the indigenous population not being able to access telehealth treatment services. Another structural barrier that has been reported to prevent the indigenous communities from accessing Mental Health services (Goetz et al., 2022).

Stigma and shame associated with mental health also prevent the indigenous community from seeking help for mental health conditions. The stigma associated with mental health by indigenous people includes the belief that mental illness is not accepted by these societies, avoidance of people who have mental health, and fear of being judged. Self-stigma, which is internalised stigma, which includes the perception of feeling weak, shameful of themselves, and embarrassed when asking for help, also keeps them from seeking help for mental health concerns. Studies have shown that participants' worry about being called crazy as well as feeling inferior prevents them from seeking help. Other than personal shame participants also worry about disgracing their families. They also fear their confidentiality and privacy being breached as their communities are small and tight-knit where everyone knows one another and people tend to "blab things" (Goetz et al., 2022).

Lack of knowledge is also one of the major factors. Indigenous people emphasise culture and their preference for mental health workers and treatment. Some of them even report not trusting indigenous providers and identify white privilege as one of the barriers to the relationship between the service provider and the indigenous client. They also have a fear of being removed from their home by the government and being placed in a mental health institute. Lack of indigenous professionals and being treated by professionals who are not from their community results and them feeling not understood. Having access to counselors from their own community helps them feel more secure and understood as it ensures cultural appropriateness. Lastly, another factor that prevents these communities from seeking help is related to the reluctance to use the formal service and their mistrust of the mainstream service (Goetz et al., 2022).

CONCLUSION

Overall as compared to the non-indigenous population, mental health is worse in the Indigenous population. This may be a result of many factors such as lack of education, fear of stigma as well as lack of services and opportunities. Therefore, it is extremely important to come up with strategies to help promote mental health in these communities. Strategies such as promoting education, reducing stigma, and introducing policies must be implemented to help support these communities.

REFERENCES

Arriagada, P., Hahmann, T., & O'Donnell, V. (2020, June 23). Indigenous people and mental health during the COVID-19 pandemic. Retrieved December 4, 2022, from https://www150.statcan.gc.ca/n1/pub/45-28-0001/2020001/article/00035-eng.htm

Bombay, A., McQuaid, R. J., Schwartz, F., Thomas, A., Anisman, H., & Matheson, K. (2018). Suicidal thoughts and attempts in First Nations communities: Links to parental indian residential school attendance across development. Journal of Developmental Origins of Health and Disease, 10(1), 123–131. https://doi.org/10.1017/s2040174418000405

Centers for Disease Control and Prevention. (2021, June 28). About mental health. Centers for Disease Control and Prevention. Retrieved December 4, 2022, from https://www.cdc.gov/mentalhealth/learn/index.htm

Corrado, R. R., & Cohen, I. M. (2003). Mental Health Profiles for a sample of British Columbia's aboriginal survivors of the Canadian Residential School System: Prepared for the Aboriginal Healing Foundation. Aboriginal Healing Foundation.

Goetz, C. J., Mushquash, C. J., & Maranzan, K. A. (2022). An integrative review of barriers and facilitators associated with mental health help seeking among indigenous populations. Psychiatric Services. https://doi.org/10.1176/appi.ps.202100503

Government of Canada, S. C. (2022, September 21). Indigenous population continues to grow and is much younger than the non-indigenous population, although the pace of growth has slowed. The Daily - . Retrieved December 6, 2022, from https://www150.statcan.gc.ca/n1/daily-quotidien/220921/dq220921a-eng.htm?indid=329 90-1&indgeo=0

Government of Canada; Indigenous Services Canada. (2022, July 9). Mental health and wellness in First Nations and Inuit communities. Government of Canada; Indigenous Services Canada. Retrieved December 4, 2022, from https://www.sac-isc.gc.ca/eng/1576089278958/1576089333975

Graham, S., Stelkia, K., Wieman, C., & Adams, E. (2021). Mental health interventions for first nation, Inuit, and Métis peoples in Canada: A systematic review. International
Indigenous Policy Journal, 12(2), 1–31. https://doi.org/10.18584/iipj.2021.12.2.10820

Kirmayer, L. J., Brass, G. M., & Tait, C. L. (2000). The Mental Health of Aboriginal Peoples:Transformations of identity and community. The Canadian Journal of Psychiatry, 45(7), 607–616. https://doi.org/10.1177/070674370004500702

Kirmayer, L. J., Brass, G. M., & Tait, C. L. (2000). The Mental Health of Aboriginal Peoples: Transformations of identity and community. The Canadian Journal of Psychiatry, 45(7), 607–616. https://doi.org/10.1177/070674370004500702

MacMillan, H. L., MacMillan, A. B., Offord, D. R., & Dingle, J. L. (1996). Aboriginal health. CMAJ : Canadian Medical Association journal = journal de l'Association medicale canadienne, 155(11), 1569–1578.

Mental illness and addiction: Facts and statistics. CAMH. (n.d.). Retrieved December 4, 2022, rom https://www.camh.ca/en/driving-change/the-crisis-is-real/mental-health-statistics

Morton Ninomiya, M., George, N., George, J., Linklater, R., Bull, J., Plain, S., Graham, K., Bernards, S., Peach, L., Stergiopoulos, V., Kurdyak, P., McKinley, G., Donnelly, P., & Wells, S. (2020). A community-driven and evidence-based approach to developing mental wellness strategies in First Nations: A program protocol. Research Involvement and Engagement, 6(1). https://doi.org/10 .1186/s40900-020-0176-9

Residential schools. Manitoba Trauma Information and Education Center. (n.d.). Retrieved December 7, 2022, from https://trauma-informed.ca/trauma-and-first-nations-people/residential-schools/#:~:text= Because%20the%20impacts%20 of%20residential,continue%20to%20permeate%20Cana dian%20society

Sikorski, C., Leatherdale, S., & Cooke, M. (2019). Tobacco, alcohol and marijuana use among indigenous youth attending off-reserve schools in Canada: Cross-sectional results from the Canadian student tobacco, alcohol and drugs survey. Health Promotion and Chronic Disease Prevention in Canada, 39(6/7), 207–215. https://doi.org/10.24095/hpcdp.39.6/7.01

Tee-Melegrito , R. A., White, M. A., & Felman , A. (2022). Mental health: Definition, common disorders, early signs, and more. Medical News Today. Retrieved December 4, 2022, from https://www.medicalnewstoday.com/articles/154543

WHO. (2022). Mental health: Strengthening our response. World Health Organization. Retrieved December 4, 2022, from https://www.who.int/news-room/fact-sheets/detail/mental-health-strengthening-our-response

INTERGENERATIONAL TRAUMA AND THE EFFECTS OF RESIDENTIAL SCHOOLS ON INDIGENOUS PEOPLE IN CANADA TODAY

By Michael Owanga

INTRODUCTION

This chapter focuses on past legislation and policies that directly affected Indigenous Canadians in the past and the impacts that they have had on their descendants today. The concept of intergenerational trauma is explained in the context of how Indigenous Canadians are currently experiencing it as a result of The Indian Act, residential schools, and the Sixties Scoop.

WHAT IS INTERGENERATIONAL TRAUMA?

Canada has a long history of committing injustices against its indigenous population. The effects of these injustices are felt not only by the victims themselves but as well as their descendants. The concept of intergenerational trauma refers to passing down the by-products of traumatic experiences (stress, depression, anxiety, etc.) down family lines. The transgenerational effects are not only psychological but familial, social, cultural, neurobiological, and possibly even genetic (DeAngelis, 2019). This passed-down trauma results from the younger generations inheriting the habits, beliefs, and practices of their predecessors. Seeing as all of these can be shaped by experiences, it makes sense that going through something traumatic can affect the way that individuals navigate the world, which they can pass on to their offspring. In regards to the First Nations people of Canada, we can see that they experience intergenerational trauma by acknowledging that most of the problems that they face today (poverty, food insecurity, mental health issues, addictions, etc.) are a result of the past experiences of their ancestors, such as residential schools and the Sixties Scoop.

Residential schools are the main attribute of the intergenerational trauma that indigenous Canadians face today. Residential schools were an attempt by the Canadian government to absolve its Indian problem[4] which sought to assimilate indigenous people towards their western ideals by removing indigenous culture from Canada. This was done by taking children as young as 5 years old from their families and bringing them to boarding schools, where they were separated from their culture and made to take on that of Europeans. The schools provided a substandard education and taught native children to be ashamed of their languages, cultural beliefs, and traditions (DeAngelis, 2019). This program which lasted over a century ended fewer than 3 decades ago and subjected children to physical, mental, and sexual abuse. They were stripped of their languages and heritage, which led to a loss of culture due to the parents' inability to pass the tradition onto their children. Underfed and malnourished, the students were particularly vulnerable to diseases such as tuberculosis and influenza (Miller, 2021). Since these children were subjected to trauma and limited displays of love during their upbringing, most became susceptible to treating their children with little affection and neglect once they grew older. These attempts at forced assimilation have failed, in part due to the resilience and resistance of many Indigenous communities (Kirmayer 2011). Although the resilience of First Nations people in Canada brought forth the preservation of their culture, the effects of the trauma that these children experienced can still be felt by indigenous populations today.

Sharon Shorty demonstrates the resilience of Canada's First Nations people well by how she navigates parenthood as a victim of intergenerational trauma. Her mother, Winnie Peterson, attended Baptist Mission School in Yukon where she was separated from her family and suffered various forms of abuse. Sharon recounts that there was little affection in her home during her childhood and that

---

4   The Indian problem refers to the view that Indigenous Canadian culture needed to be eradicated in order to ensure unity within the country.

she struggled to show affection to her son years later (Shorty, 2018). This confused her, but it all made sense to her when she grew older and learned that her parents had been taken away from their families and did not experience much parental affection during their respective upbringings. She noticed parallels between how she was treated as a child and how she had been treating her son and sought to break the cycle by healing. One method she used to seek reconciliation was attending events held for survivors of residential schools and hearing their stories and how their experiences affected their lives as adults. At one of these events, a birthday party was held for the survivors to acknowledge that their birthdays had never been celebrated in residential schools (Shorty, 2018). This made her realise why on her birthdays she had barely had any birthday parties growing up and that it was important to have birthday parties for her son (Shorty, 2018). Sharon's story demonstrates that the impacts of residential schools are showing up later on with varying levels of significance, from not celebrating birthdays to not showing affection. These all have to do with child neglect and the impacts that it can have on future generations. We can also learn from Sharon that to mend what is broken, it is important to learn from the mistakes of the past to seek reconciliation and healing.

Many children experienced psychological, spiritual, physical, and sexual abuse at the hands of their so-called caregivers in the residential school system (Menzies, 2020). Once these children grew into adulthood, they were left without an appropriate point of reference for how adults were supposed to treat children. Many survivors of residential schools weren't able to form lifelong bonds with their parents, as they spent most of their lives separated from them. This led to a difference in culture, values, and in some cases a language barrier, which all prevented these people from getting to know their parents. Eventually, these survivors would also have to go through losing their children to this system, which separated them from familial affection even more. Without a support system, many survivors turned to substance abuse in an attempt to remove themselves from the trauma that they had experienced. We can also attribute poverty to the higher rates of substance abuse in indigenous communities. The substandard education provided in residential schools led to chronic unemployment or underemployment (Wolastoqiyik, 2020). This led to a snowball effect, where the survivors of these schools were left to fend for themselves in the streets where drug use was rampant, with nobody looking out for them, they made use of a readily available means of escape.

WHAT ELSE CONTRIBUTES TO THE INTERGENERATIONAL TRAUMA OF INDIGENOUS PEOPLE?

Residential schools were not the only method that the Canadian government used to get rid of its Indian problem. The Sixties Scoop was also implemented as a means to further separate Indigenous children from their heritage. Beginning in the 1950s and going into the 80s, the purpose of the Sixties Scoop was to separate Indigenous newborns and young children from their birth homes to be adopted into white families from all over Canada, the United States, and in some cases, parts of Europe and Australasia. This was done in order to leave the adoptees with a lost sense of cultural identity (Sinclair, 2020). The removal of these children from their homes to be placed into the welfare system was unethical because it was unnecessary. These children were well cared for and were not in any danger at home. The Canadian government came up with this system as a way to bypass having to deal with Indigenous child-welfare issues such as poverty and food insecurity. At the time, social workers did not need permission from local authorities to remove children from their homes, which led to roughly 20,000 Indigenous children being "scooped" with little to no justification. The Sixties Scoop was an extension of paternalistic policies in Canada that sought the assimilation of Indigenous cultures and communities (Sinclair, 2020). The Sixties Scoop came to an end following the passing of the Child, Family, and Community Services Act in 1980, which made it mandatory for social workers to consult band councils before removing an Indigenous child from the community. Although the Sixties Scoop came to an end, the overrepresentation of Indigenous youth in the Canadian foster care system remains rampant today.

We can directly attribute First Nations children being the highest demographic group in the foster care system today to the Sixties Scoop. Although legislation and laws that prevent Indigenous youth from being taken away from their families unjustifiably have been set in place, the culture of social welfare workers vying to separate indigenous children from their families has not gone away. Birth alerts refer to a system where social workers request the hospital staff to notify them once expectant mothers give birth because they believe that the baby is at risk (Morgan, 2021). This practice disproportionately affects Indigenous women and redesigns Canada's racist policies (ie. Sixties Scoop) of the past in a way that allows them to exist today. We saw an example of this when an apprehension order was given to an Indigenous Calgary mother 4 days after giving birth to her son in January 2013. This meant that her newborn would be taken into government custody under false pretences that she was unfit to care for the child. According to the notes of the social worker on the case, the woman (who had been a minor at the time) had some experiences with domestic violence and sexual abuse at her mother's house, where she did not live (Morgan, 2021). The society knew about this because the mother, "Cora" had previously reached out for resources to remove herself from the situation, but did not receive any. It is speculated that the reasoning for this is from some internal bias of the social worker due to notes such as "Several sexual assaults have happened to her since she was 15 including [...] a man who raped her [...] at her mother's home.[...] however continued to return to her mother's home under these occurrences" (Morgan, 2021). That same social worker applied for an apprehension order after hearing that Cora was pregnant due to the risks of domestic violence. Background checks indicate that Cora was living with her partner and his cousin at the time and was removed from the abusers of her past (Morgan, 2021). Cora, whose real name is being withheld, went through some parenting classes and social programs and eventually reunited with her son. Despite making up only 5% of the population in Canada, Indigenous people make up 53.8% in foster care (StatsCan, 2022). Stories like that of Cora are common for Indigenous women in Canada and are reminiscent of the occurrences of the Sixties Scoop.

The trauma that the victims of the Sixties Scoop went through is immense and the impacts of that trauma still affect them in their adult lives. Most children grew up without being educated about their birth cultures, which led to feelings of shame, loneliness, and confusion (Sinclair, 2020). Although some of the children did get adopted into loving families, most of these families weren't able to provide the children with knowledge about their culture. This resulted in the Indigenous adoptees growing up to become adults who felt lost and alone in the world. In order for birth records to be opened, both the birth parents and the separated children would have to consent, which meant that reunions typically didn't happen for decades. Some adoptees have since come forward and mentioned being subjected to various forms of abuse under the care of their adoptive families. As a result of the negative impacts of the experiences of adoptees during the Sixties Scoop, class action lawsuits have opened up against the governments of Ontario, Manitoba, Saskatchewan, and Alberta (Sinclair, 2021).

WHAT IS THE TRUTH AND RECONCILIATION COMMISSION?

The Truth and Reconciliation Commission refers to a program set in place by the Canadian government to reconcile survivors of residential schools and their families. This means that the Canadian government is making amends with the Indigenous community on account of the injustices that they have imposed on First Nations communities over the years (ie. residential schools, Sixties Scoop). The Truth and Reconciliation Commission was introduced in June 2008 through a legal settlement between The Canadian Federal government and the First Nations, Inuit, and Métis peoples of Canada. The TRC's mandate was to inform all Canadians about what happened in residential schools. The TRC documents the truth of anyone personally affected by the residential school experience (Truth and Reconciliation Commission of Canada, n.d.). The TRC has also brought forth 94 calls to action, which are meant to inform Canadians on how they can aid Indigenous communities in the healing process, most notably by acknowledging the full history of the residential school system, thereby preventing anything similar from happening again in Canada's future. The aim of the calls to action is to have Canadian citizens understand the full scale and severity of the long-lasting effects of the residential school system and how they still affect indigenous communities today, which is intended to lead to reconciliation.

Kevin Lamoureux refers to the 94 Calls to Action as a roadmap home. What he means by this is that the Calls to Action act as an outline for Canada to orient itself in the direction of where we could be today if Indigenous people hadn't suffered injustices in the past. The Calls to Action do benefit Indigenous Canadians, especially since the Calls to Action were designed by Indigenous people themselves. By engaging non-Indigenous and Indigenous communities in Canada to acknowledge the horrific practices that went on in residential schools, the process of reconciliation becomes more practical in the sense that more people will understand the gravity of the situation and prevent anything similar from happening again in the future. Another benefit of the Calls to Action is their intended impact on the Indigenous workforce. Call Number 92, entitled Business and Reconciliation, recommends to the corporate sector in Canada to adopt the United Nations on the Rights of Indigenous Peoples and apply its core principles involving the lands and resources of Indigenous peoples (*TRC Call to Action*, n.d.). This would mean that any economic development projects taking place on Indigenous land would require the informed and prior consent of Indigenous peoples. This would benefit Indigenous Canadians by allowing them to dictate what happens to their land, as well as non-Indigenous Canadians via its implications on sustainable development, that being the prevention of projects that would cause habit loss and/ or the burning of fossil fuels, such as building pipelines. The Bussiness and Reconciliation Call also recommends that Indigenous Canadians have equitable access to jobs, training, and education opportunities in the corporate sector, which is aimed to tackle the disproportionate rates of poverty that Indigenous communities face in Canada (*TRC Call to Action*, n.d.).

Progress on the implementation of the Truth and Reconciliation Calls to action has been quite slow. Having been introduced in 2015, only 12 of 94 have been completed as of December 2022. The main reason for this is that some require the Canadian Federal government to use resources, such as money, which it can't do all at once. Progress is being made, however, it isn't easy to implement every Call to Action immediately. CTA Number 1 (in progress) concerns the reduction of Indigenous in the Canadian foster care system. This Call to Action requires resources to be provided to Indigenous communities and cultural competence training for social workers. Additionally, the government is working with Indigenous community leaders to reform the child welfare system in Canada (Reconciliation, n.d.). The Canadian Federal Government has not, however, made any recent attempts to amend/ abolish The Indian Act. The Indian Act is the main form of legislation in Canada whose purpose was to assimilate Indigenous populations into Euro-Canadian society by outlining governmental obligations to First Nations peoples (Parrott, 2022). This Act was responsible for making attendance at residential schools mandatory to further the Canadian government's goal to assimilate its First Nations peoples. The Indian Act made it illegal for First Nations people to practise their culture publicly. This meant that First Nations people couldn't speak their languages, wear traditional clothing or hold any celebrations in their communities. Having first been introduced in 1876, the Indian Act was amended in 1951, following the second world war. The amendment allowed women to be included in band council elections, which they were barred from prior. Band councils refer to a group of elected officials made of chiefs and other executives in First Nations communities. The original Indian Act facilitated the absolution of hereditary chiefs, who gained their positions by birthright and replaced them with band councils. Another by-product of the Indian Act was the Pass System, which restricted the movement of Indigenous people off reserves. These restrictive policies have had lasting impacts on generations of Indigenous people, as restrictions on mobility caused damage to Indigenous economies, cultures, and societies (Parrott, 2022).

The Indian Act was amended and given royal assent[5] in 1951. The changes removed the cultural restrictions of the original Indian Act, such as the right to have public ceremonies, speak Indigenous languages, and do traditional dances in public. This amendment did not mean that the Indian Act was no longer discriminatory.

5   Royal assent refers to a bill being passed by the House of Parliament

Following the amendment of 1951, provincial governments were given control over the child welfare system, which led to the Sixties Scoop (Parrott, 2022). The Indian Act was also still responsible for Indigenous Canadians not having the right to vote without losing their status. Another amendment came in 1985, which pertained to the absolution of The Indian Act's discrimination against women, following The United Nations Human Rights Commission ruling that Canada was in violation of Article 27 of the International Covenant on Civil and Political Rights by revoking the status of Indigenous women (Parrott, 2022). Despite amendments being made over the years, the Indian Act still affects Indigenous communities today in terms of politics, economics, and culture through the intergenerational trauma that it caused through residential schools and the prohibition of practicing culture.

CONCLUSION

Many of the problems that Indigenous people in Canada face today, such as disproportionate levels of poverty, unemployment, overrepresentation in the welfare system, and substance abuse issues are a result of jurisdictions imposed on their ancestors following the Indian Act of 1876. Residential schools prevented generations of Indigenous children from learning about their heritage and separated them from their families, causing most to grow into adults who didn't know anything about knew very little about their heritage. The substandard education that they received in these facilities meant that they had fewer employment opportunities than their non-Indigenous counterparts, which led to poverty for many survivors to end up on the streets. The Truth and Reconciliation Commission has provided 94 Calls to Action, which encourage the Canadian government to make amends with the Indigenous communities by implementing policies that aid towards healing. The idea of this is that it will encourage Canadians to acknowledge what happened in the past, thereby preventing anything similar from ever happening again in the future.

REFERENCES

DeAngelis, T. (2019, February 1). The legacy of trauma. Monitor on Psychology, 50(2). https://www.apa.org/monitor/2019/02/legacy-trauma

Kirmayer LJ, Dandeneau S, Marshall E, Phillips MK, Williamson KJ. Rethinking Resilience from Indigenous Perspectives. The Canadian Journal of Psychiatry. 2011;56(2):84-91. doi:10.1177/070674371105600203

Menzies, P. (2020). Intergenerational Trauma and Residential Schools. In The Canadian Encyclopedia. Retrieved from https://www.thecanadianencyclopedia.ca/en/article/intergenerational-trauma-and-resident ial-schools

Shorty, S. (2018, November 4). There are thousands of intergenerational survivors' stories — this is mine. CBC. Retrieved December 3, 2022, from https://www.cbc.ca/news/canada/north/intergenerational-survivor-residential-school-shar on-shorty-1.4878247

Sinclair, N., & Dainard, S. (2020). Sixties Scoop. In The Canadian Encyclopedia. Retrieved from https://www.thecanadianencyclopedia.ca/en/article/sixties-scoop

The Daily — Indigenous population continues to grow and is much younger than the non-Indigenous population, although the pace of growth has slowed. (2022, September 21). Statistique Canada. Retrieved December 3, 2022, from https://www150.statcan.gc.ca/n1/daily-quotidien/220921/dq220921a-eng.htm

TRC Call to Action. (n.d.). Indigenous Works. Retrieved December 4, 2022, fromhttps://indigenousworks.ca/en/partnership/what-does-intersection-mean/trc-call-action

Wolastoqiyik. (2020, April 3). Wolastoqiyik Family Services - Fredericton. Retrieved November 20, 2022, from https://www.wfsnb.ca/post/the-impact-of-residential-schools

CHAPTER 6

THE ROLES AND RELATIONSHIPS BETWEEN ANIMALS AND INDIGENOUS PEOPLE

By Ryan Doleweerd

INTRODUCTION

This chapter will explore the roles of animals in the lives of Indigenous people from around the world, both past and present. In this line of investigation, one will learn about how the lives of Indigenous people and the animals in their own respective regions are intertwined, and as a result will understand why the Indigenous people value the importance of a good relationship with animals.

Indigenous people as defined by the Canadian Government is an inclusive name for the original people of North America and their descendants. There are three recognized groups of Indigenous people: The First Nations, Inuit, and Métis people. Each group of people has their own unique history, languages, practices, and spiritual beliefs (Government of Canada, 2022).

Animals are deeply ingrained into the fabric of the lives of Indigenous people. Indigenous people have a fundamentally closer relationship to animals as they have lived among animals much longer than any other people (Legge & Robinson, 2017). Many Indigenous cultures consider animals to hold importance similar to that of human beings. Animals have unique roles as knowledge-holders due to their history in their habitat and knowledge of it. To Indigenous persons, animals can be symbolic and play key roles in shared stories, but they are also predators, prey, and a unique species. As they are living creatures, their lives are of value and deserve dignity (Weatherdon, 2022). Overall, a consensus that carries through the Indigenous culture is the idea that this relationship is reciprocal. As long as the relationship is honoured by both parties, humans will have food and materials, and animals are treated respectfully by humans, ensuring their survival as a species (Zdor, 2009).

ANIMALS IN INDIGENOUS CULTURE

Animals have multiple roles within Indigenous culture, from stories to ceremonies.There are many stories within Indigenous cultures that involve animals (Forbes, 2001). Many of these stories often involve animals that can talk, think, and live as humans do. Not to be mistaken with anthropomorphism (the attribution of human characteristics or behaviour onto a non-human entity), they view it as the animals undergoing personhood, which is common to all lifeforms (Legge & Robinson, 2017). The purpose of these stories is to communicate different ideas onto the listener. These tales have many different purposes, to share important geological or historical information or moral, ethical and religious ideals (Weatherdon, 2022). This kinship can be taken further however, as some Indigenous traditions, which are more commonly found within Inuit communities, believe that people can transform from human to animal. This is depicted in many stories where a human eventually transforms into some sort of animal, intentional or inadvertently. This is because it is believed that the boundary between the physical and spiritual worlds, and the boundary between life forms like humans, animals and plants, can be easily crossed. This is to show as Indigenous belief is so strong and their interconnectedness with animals is great that transformation from human into animal can occur. However, it is less common for an animal to transform into a human as they are more likely to just take on human attributes (Legge & Robinson, 2017).

One large component of many Indigenous cultures is ceremonies, songs, and dance. It is very common for regional animals of specific Indigenous communities to be featured in songs or central to the ceremonies and dances. For the Yupik and Chukchi peoples in the region that is now part of northern Russia, the polar bear is a very common animal in their celebrations and legends (Zdor, 2009). To them and the Inuits in northern Canada, the polar bear has a large role in their culture as it provides plentiful materials like fur, meat, and bones. As well, until these northern Indigenous communities had firearms, the polar bear was the other primary predator alongside the Inuit in the region. This shows that for most of the Inuit polar bear relationship, polar bears were fairly equal to the Inuit, so understandably their role in the Inuit culture would be very impactful (Wenzel, 2004).

ANIMALS IN INDIGENOUS COMMUNITIES VERSUS TREATMENT IN SETTLER CULTURE

Settler culture, which is largely based on Christian values, has the Creation story in the book of Genesis which puts a hierarchy of firstly God, then humans, animals, and plants at the bottom (Weatherdon, 2022). This can be understood as a direct conflict in ideals, Indigenous people place a much higher value on animal life (Legge & Robinson, 2017). Most Indigenous practices are the root of believing in animism. Animism is the attribution of all things having a soul, whether that be plants, animals or even inanimate objects (Forbes, 2001). Many Indigenous creation stories describe humans as the younger sibling to animals. The Indigenous people's value of life is often all-encompassing and is much more sensitive to the roles of animals in our world in comparison to Christian settlers in the west. These settlers historically viewed themselves as greater than animals, with their survival being much more important (Legge & Robinson, 2017). Indigenous people value animal life, and do not take any life for granted which is due to their close ties to animals and beliefs about animals. Indigenous people want to live harmoniously with animals and nature, using only resources that are needed and using all parts of the animal as they respect its life and its death so they can eat (Weatherdon, 2022). Due to this large gap in animal treatment and the views of the Indigenous people, there are treaties that allow Indigenous people to hunt certain animals that may be endangered or on watch (Zdor, 2009). Polar bear meat and fur is an important resource for those Inuit communities. It provides the Inuit with food, the fur can be used for their clothing, bedding, or sold at auctions, and the bones can be used for carving (Wong & Murphy, 2016). Hence, the Inuit have been given permission by a treaty to hunt polar bears within certain limits. This means the Indigenous people can both survive in the harsh climate easier and there is less risk of polar bears becoming extinct (Zdor, 2009). Currently, one concern of Indigenous people is the portrayal of their hunting practices by governments. They portray Indigenous hunting practices to be causing risk to many species when that is not the case (Gadamus & Raymond-Yakoubian, 2015). The Indigenous people take only what they need, so it is the western civilization projecting their own habits onto Indigenous people which is not true (Weatherdon, 2022).

RESPECTING ANIMAL LIFE

For Indigenous people they view animals, plants and ecosystems as having value to both humans, but to other different parts of the ecosystem. They understand that the balance of the ecosystem must be maintained so all species can thrive. Abuse to the ecosystem can throw it out of balance and result in the collapse of the ecosystem (Weatherdon, 2022). Up north where walrus and seal hunting occur, the Indigenous people have many issues with Western hunting practices. They find Western hunting practices disturb the environment. Tribe leaders and Indigenous hunters have found the noise and pollution due to industrial fishing to do much harm to the region. They believe the government should be doing more to protect these animals being overfished (Gadamus & Raymond-Yakoubian, 2015). This respect stems from their strong belief that there is a sacredness in all life, whether it be animal or human (Dell et al., 2008). As this is a mutually reciprocal relationship, if other parties cause issues with the human and animal relationship, the relationship Indigenous people have with the animals in their regions will be damaged as a result of this, which the Indigenous people do not want (Zdor, 2009).

INDIGENOUS THERAPY AND ANIMALS

In recent years there has been an increase in animal assisted therapy. However, the horse and other equines are most commonly used when working with Indigenous youth. One issue that affects Indigenous youth is volatile solvent abuse. Volatile solvent abuse is to intentionally inhale aerosols and volatile solvents like gasoline and solvents found in glue. One way that is being used to help treat the solvent abuse problem in youth, is equine assisted learning. Though equine assisted learning can also be used to help treat other mental health, addictions, behavioural, and emotional issues facing youth, it is most commonly used in treating Indigenous youth with volatile solvent abuse issues (Dell et al., 2008).

The horse has had a large role in Indigenous culture since it was introduced by the Spanish and understanding its role in Indigenous culture is paramount in the It is commonly used when hunting and gathering, and plays a significant part in many ceremonies, like one that is aptly named the Horse Dance. The idea that the horse is a sort of truth teller and is believed that when used in the therapy it will guide these misguided youth each back onto their own right path (Dell et al., 2008). The horse's spirit is said to help people understand their place in the circle of life. This understanding of one's place, is a critical foundation to positive health. As it is said that horses assist spiritually, the horse will help the individual working with it in therapy, as connection with the horse helps repair the spiritual connection the youth may have been missing (Chalmers & Dell, 2011). This horse assisted healing program works by using the horse to teach these struggling individuals life skills and positive learning practices. This type of program is an educational program that uses direct experiences and contact with a horse to address emotional and behavioural issues facing each individual (Dell et al., 2011). In most cases, horse assisted learning is done in group and focuses on ground activities rather teaching the struggling youth about horse riding. However, there has been an increase in therapeutic programs focused towards horseback riding (Dell et al., 2008). Riding or non-riding programs, the commonality is the developing bond between the youth and the horse. It is based on deep trust, and as some past participants describe how they feel the horse believed in them. As the participant worked on their own issues the horse would trust the participant more and more. The participant learns transferable skills from horse to human as they develop their relationship with the horse. These skills included patience and leadership, as well as verbal and non-verbal communication. It meant they learned to read the body language of the horses, which is helpful in learning to communicate better with others as they pay attention to the body language of other people. The youth gained confidence as they improved the skills they were learning so they could have a closer bond with the horse. This therapy was also effective in showing the youth positive role models. This came in the form of the staff who took care of the horses. They showed the youth what it was like to care about something, to be responsible, and gave them a positive role model they could work towards. All because of the trust the horses had in the staff, and the bond between the staff and the horses. Overall, this therapy has had resounding effects on the wellbeing of Indigenous youth, all because of the bond between human and animal and was compounded by their Indigenous backgrounds that place humans and animals as equals (Dell et al., 2011).

ATTACKS ON INDIGENOUS PEOPLE AND ANIMALS

Both animals and Indigenous people have been victims of colonial violence. The assaults on animals may also be considered attacks on Indigenous persons because of the close relationships they hold with their environment and animals within it. When settlers first came to North America, they would kill many animals for food which was the case for the plains buffalo (Weatherdon, 2022), or like the beaver which was hunted for its fur. The beaver was highly sought after in the area that is now Canada as its fur was the most highly prized of the animals in the region (Daschuk, 2012). This impacted both the ecosystem, and the ability of the Indigenous people to find food and get materials. When the plains buffalo were slaughtered by the colonisers, it resulted in roughly one quarter of the Indigenous people in that area starving to death. It was very easy for the settlers to kill the plains buffalo as they had access to guns, so it quickly became a mass killing of plains buffalo. Some of the mass killings of animals was intentionally meant to limit the food supply of the Indigenous people in line with other genocidal practices (Weatherdon, 2022). As the beaver was hunted across the now Canadian prairies by settlers, it resulted in clearing out the entire beaver population from the area. It is now why beavers are now found infrequently in the prairies (Daschuk, 2012).

Currently there are a number of Indigenous tribes working with governments to revitalise populations of animals. In 1991, the Intertribal Buffalo Council was formed. This council based out of the United States includes 58 tribes and 19 states. The goal of the council is to restore and nurture the bison populations as a result of what happened to the bison populations as a result of western colonisation. These population restorations can be seen as a rejuvenation religiously too. As they restore populations, they perform ceremonies, learn about different species, all in the hope to fix the damaged relationship between humans and animals that was caused by overhunting commonly by the western settlers (Weatherdon, 2022).

Another type of attack on the Indigenous people and animals came from domesticated animals brought by settlers. These animals carried diseases that hurt many Indigenous populations and many species of animals. These animals also disturbed the ecosystems they settled in. They scared off many animals residing in the areas, or the settlers would settle in an area which disturbed the habitat of those native animals. This resulted in much more difficulty for the Indigenous people as finding the animals was more difficult as many hunting practices were no longer viable due to the disturbances. One other large disturbance was the deliberate invasion of the settlers with their domesticated animals onto Indigenous reserve lands to graze. All of these attacks resulted in the Indigenous people killing the settler's livestock for food so that they could survive (Weatherdon, 2022). These two groups, animals and Indigenous people, had experiences with settlers that parallel each other, and also impacted one another. The Indigenous and the animals lost their land, food sources, felt sick to disease, and were victims of violence from settlers. None of these things happened before the settlers came because of the mutually beneficial relationship the animals and Indigenous people have (Weatherdon, 2022).

ANIMAL INFLUENCE WITHIN INDIGENOUS RELIGIONS

There is variation within Indigenous communities with the role of animals in Indigenous spirituality and religion, however a commonality is the prominent role they have within it. The prominent ways they generally appear are as historically significant creatures, as wise protectors, a part of ceremonies, and in kinship systems (Legge & Robinson, 2017).

The historical significance of animals to Indigenous people is huge. Humans can only survive where there is food. Traditionally, because animals make up a large part of the Indigenous diet, Indigenous people must settle where there are animals so they can eat. When settlers came and disturbed the ecosystem, many Indigenous communities would migrate with the animals when they moved. If the food source moves away, the only option was to follow the food source or risk starvation (Legge & Robinson, 2017).

They are wise protectors because these animals have been so successful at surviving in their ecosystem. There is much that can be learned from animals as they guide and teach about their habitat as they are experts at surviving in their own habitat. These animals, because they are so knowledgeable, can be seen as protectors to communities and individuals. This is because of the knowledge they share (Legge & Robinson, 2017).

The role of animals in ceremonies has large variations. A person may embody an animal through dance. This is especially common in hunting rituals. They do these hunting rituals to honour the animals, because by living alongside animals respectfully will mean there will always be animals reproducing, and always enough food to survive (Legge & Robinson, 2017).

Other ceremonies or dances are particularly focused on an animal for different reasons. One time to welcome back the people who fought in World War II, some Indigenous communities put on a horse dance (Dell et al., 2008). One of those communities was Muskoday First Nations who are located in the area that is near Prince Albert, Saskatchewan. This is just one example of how animals are used in ceremonies (White Buffalo Treatment Centre, n.d.).

This animal-human kinship has been manifested largely into commonly used Indigenous cultural expressions. These expressions took the form of animal clans and totems. It is very common for an Indigenous person to have the last name of an animal that is significant. During ceremonies the animal skin is worn as part of regalia identifying their clan or family (Legge & Robinson, 2017).

One example of the role of animals within some Indigenous religions is the doodem. For the Anishnaabeg people, the doodem is a kinship system that places animals and humans in an interdependent relationship. This tradition comes from a creation story involving great non-humanlike creatures (Weatherdon, 2022). These are viewed as holy and animal-like creatures (Forbes, 2001). They also believe they have two souls. One soul can go to the afterlife, the other soul is shared with the doodem, as the doodem has a soul. These doodem are also associated with certain traits (Weatherdon, 2022). The horse is viewed as a sort of teller of truth (Dell et al., 2008). The bear is shown as representing strength and courage (Weatherdon, 2022). These symbolic animal views from their religion play many roles in day to day Indigenous life.

CONCLUSION

It is clear that the relationship with animals is invaluable to Indigenous people which is evident by their deep relationship with them. Animals and Indigenous people have such an intertwined history that animals have become such a huge part of the Indigenous culture (Weatherdon, 2022). The respect that the Indigenous people show the animals is a direct result of their deep relationship with them. This relationship shows that these two groups are highly interdependent on each other and have a huge role in the lives of each other. This relationship is built on mutual respect and mutual benefit. If either party does not respect the other, the relationship would collapse and cause major problems for both parties, as both gain something from this relationship which would be lost (Zdor, 2009).

REFERENCES

Chalmers, D., & Dell, C. A. (2011). Equine-Assisted Therapy with First Nations Youth in Residential Treatment for Volatile Substance Misuse: Building an Empirical Knowledge Base. Native Studies Review, 20(1).

Daschuk, J. (2012). Who Killed the Prairie Beaver? an environmental Case for eighteenth Century migration in Western Canada. Prairie Forum, 37, 151–172.

Dell, C. A., Chalmers, D., Bresette, N., Swain, S., Rankin, D., & Hopkins, C. (2011). A healing space: The experiences of First Nations and Inuit youth with equine-assisted learning (EAL). Child & Youth Care Forum, 40(4), 319–336. https://doi.org/10.1007/s10566-011-9140-z

Dell, C. A., Dell, D., Sauve, E., & MacKinnon, T. (2008). Horse as Healer: An Examination of Equine Assisted Learning in the Healing of First Nations Youth from Solvent Abuse. In D. Chalmers (Ed.), Pimatisiwin: A Journal of Aboriginal and Indigenous Community Health (1st ed., Vol. 6, pp. 81–106). essay, Native Counselling Services of Alberta.

Forbes, J. D. (2001). Indigenous Americans: Spirituality and Ecos. Daedalus, 130(4), 283. https://link.gale.com/apps/doc/A79210535/AONE?u=ocul_mcmaster&sid=bookmark-A ONE&xid=09d761f1

Gadamus, L., & Raymond-Yakoubian, J. (2015). A Bering Strait Indigenous Framework for Resource Management: Respectful Seal and Walrus Hunting. Arctic Anthropology 52(2), 87-101. https://www.muse.jhu.edu/article/612137.

Government of Canada; Crown-Indigenous Relations and Northern Affairs Canada; (2022, August 30). Indigenous peoples and communities. Government of Canada; Crown-Indigenous Relations and Northern Affairs Canada; Retrieved December 4, 2022, from https://www.rcaanc-cirnac.gc.ca/eng/1100100013785/1529102490303

Legge, M. M., & Robinson, M. (2017). Animals in Indigenous Spiritualities: Implications for Critical Social Work. Journal of INDIGENOUS SOCIAL DEVELOPMENT, 6(1). Weatherdon, M. S. (2022). Religion, animals, and indigenous traditions. Religions, 13(7), 654. https://doi.org/10.3390/rel13070654

Wenzel, G. W. (2004). Polar Bear as a Resource: An Overview.

White Buffalo Treatment Centre. (n.d.). Retrieved December 4, 2022, from https://www.wbtc.ca/

Wong, P. B. Y., & Murphy, R. W. (2016). Inuit methods of identifying polar bear characteristics:Potential for Inuit inclusion in polar bear surveys + supplementary appendix tables S1 to S5 (see article tools). ARCTIC, 69(4), 406. https://doi.org/10.14430/arctic4605

Zdor, E. (2009). Traditional knowledge about polar bear in Chukotka. Études/Inuit/Studies, 31(1-2), 321–323. https://doi.org/10.7202/019734ar

CHAPTER 7

GENDERED IMPACTS AGAINST INDIGENOUS WOMEN AND GIRLS IN CANADA AND THE UNITED STATES

By Brianna Bedran

INTRODUCTION

In this chapter, we will be exploring the gendered impacts that colonisation and years of structural racism has on marginalised Indigenous women and girls. While colonisation is often described as a problem of the past, the impacts are long lasting and are perpetuated by existing structural factors which we will explore in this chapter that include; legislations, negligence by the criminal justice system, and socioeconomic factors that all work as forces against Indigenous women's ability to live comfortably, and safely. This chapter considers both Canada and the United States, however there is more of a focus on Canada.

Colonial harm is often further perpetuated through western academia where Indigenous women's voices are often not represented accurately and their lived experiences are disregarded (McGuire at al., 2022). Thus, the significance of this chapter is to include a mix of qualitative and quantitative information that address the importance of intersectionality in policy-making and Indigenous studies. For this chapter, the intersectionality of the obstacles of being an Indigenous and being woman is discussed. There are many great sources that have contributed to the work of this chapter, but to name a few that stand out particularly in this chapter, we would like to acknowledge the work of McGuire et al., Samuel Perreault et al., and McKenzie et al,. The information provided by these authors help greatly with the understanding of indigenous injustice, and we invite readers to take a look at their work as well to further grasp this topic.

THE INDIAN ACT AND IDENTITY ERASURE

Various forms of colonial harms have resulted in societal indifference and racism towards Indigenous women in Canada. These colonial harms have led to their own conflict with their identity, victimisation, and over-representation amongst federally incarcerated women in Canada (McGuire at al., 2022). One of the impacts of colonisation to be examined first is the Indian Act. It is important to note that negative impacts of the Indian Act do not exclude men (as well as any of the other topics explored), however for the purpose of this chapter we will only be examining the ones that have a particular influence on Indigenous women. In order to be recognized federally as Indigenous in both Canada or the United States, an individual must be able to comply with very specific standards of government regulation (Indigenous Foundations, 2009). Thus, the Indian Act in Canada signifies a lot more than simply a body of laws that for over a century now have applied stringent regulations on every part of an Indigenous person's life (Indigenous Foundations, 2009). In accordance with the description provided by Indigenous Foundations at the University of British Columbia, The Indian Act represents forms of understanding Native identity as a regulatory regime, organising a conceptual framework that has shaped contemporary Native life in ways that are now so familiar as to almost seem "natural" (Indigenous Foundations, 2009).

For many years now, patriarchal stipulations of the Indian Act that dictates who can claim their rightfully owned Indian status have had a disproportionate effect on indigenous women (Wesley, 2012) and (McGuire et al., 2022). For example, certain regulations in the Indian Act can result in federally-imposed banishment, which can possibly result in women losing their legal status as Indigenous should they choose to marry non-status men (McGuire et al., 2022). The banishing of womens Indigenous status can create space for unsafe positions such as, and not restricted to alienation, including isolation from their community, family, and culture altogether (McGuire at al., 2022) and (De Finney, 2017) and (Wesley,

2012). The regulations of the Indian Act and its cause of identity erasure have also resulted in the disempowerment of generations of Indigenous women, leading to shame and serious identity issues, intensifying their already precarious position in Canada (Amnesty International, 2008) and (McGuire et al., 2022). This bureaucratic form of loss of identity through the Indian Act erodes the important roles of Indigenous women in their communities and severely impacts Indigenous women's power and autonomy (Alfred and Corntassel, 2005) and (Amnesty International, 2008) and (McGuire at al., 2022). The sense of community is an important aspect of an Indigenous person's life-which we will be covering briefly in the third section, so for colonising bureaucratic forms to alter their sense of belonging in their own communities calls for serious attention to be paid to the Indian Act. While there are many studies that address the consequences of the Indian Act, such as the references mentioned above, not much has yet changed. Intersectionality is required for policy making and legislation regarding Indigenous affairs to seriously modify this act's impact on Indigenous women's disempowerment and unsafe position in Canada and the United States.

GOVERNMENT VIOLENCE AGAINST INDIGENOUS WOMEN

These feelings of disempowerment are important as its influence is not only on the mental health of Indigenous women, but extends to their physical well-being as well. As mentioned earlier, and supported by The National Inquiry, it is suggested that the silencing of indigenous women through a multitude of colonial measures is a major contributor to their feelings, and the reality of a lack of safety and justice Indigenous women continue to experience (2019a: 167). This lack of justice and overall safety is exacerbated by the intersection of being female and Indigenous, hence indigenous women are being subject to both racial and gendered violence (McGuire et al., 2022). Indigenous women carry the constant burden of feeling unsafe in their own communities as non-indigenous local authorities have proven to refuse to treat them as worthy of protection, which we will further examine in this section.

The law enforcement in Canada is another major, and incredibly complex force to combat the victimisation of Indigenous women in Canada (McGuire at al., 2022). Many Indigenous women in Canada have been victimized whether it is through the aforementioned statesanctioned loss of identity such as the Indian Act, as well as being subject to medical testing, being detained from their families, forced sterilization, racism, emotional, physical, and/or sexual abuse all due to their socially constructed persona as less than human. These personas are perpetuated by the government, and consequently the surrounding non-indigenous communities (McGuire at al., 2022). This criminality and victimization is situated within the persistent forces of colonialism, including their construction as having non-human bodies deemed worthy of harm, abuse, and even death (Razack, 1998)–not to mention this on top of the racism, discrimination, and marginalization they already experience (Balfour, 2008) and (De Finney, 2017) and (McGuire et al., 2022). It is here that we can really see the significance of intersectionality in the understanding of the struggles indigenous women face in the western world, as any of the obstacles they are presented with is simply on top of a multitude of all the other ones they are currently facing. These are structural barriers that call for the attention towards the fact that all the forces are working as one and make their lives more strenuous.

Indigenous women further lack safety and justice in that legal authorities have often been found to dismiss their disappearances or lack of safety despite clear evidence that would generate alarm or worry in any other non-marginalized communities. When it comes to Missing and Murdered Indigenous women and Girls (MMIWG) National Inquiry claims that "nobody is listening...nobody seems to care...there's no wrongdoing of the police in this country," as they are not held to account for their dismissal of indigenous safety (National Inquiry, 2019a: 622). The processes of dehumanization, sexualization, and control contribute to Indigenous women continuing to dissapear be murdered, or confined (McGuire et al., 2022). Furthermore, due to the lack of action taken by government and local authorities, families of MMIWG have been left with no choice but to take matters into their own hands. For example, family members are having to carry the burden of doing their own searches for their daughters in ditches, creeks, and abandoned buildings (National Inquiry, 2019a) and (McGuire et al., 2022). While the efforts taken by family and community members should certainly be acknowledged, the fact that they could not rely on their own local law enforcement represents the severity of the MMIWG crisis. Authorities' quick dismissal of their whereabouts raises serious concern for the safety of Indigenous Women. This staggering lack of accountability has resulted in worried and grieving families of MMIWG to conduct their own searches, without the necessary help and resources of authorities that would help with cases being resolved much more efficiently and quickly, providing closure for families and friends.

To further illustrate the severity of this negligence, National Inquiry describes some alarming and disturbing stories reported by Indigenous persons. Stephanie H. reported to National Inquiry that when her indigenous mother was murdered and found at the bottom of a set of stairs with blunt force trauma to the head, the couple of investigating officers were overheard making racist remarkers. The officers were overheard saying, "another drunken Indian just fell down the stairs" (National Inquiry, 2019a: 470–471). This situation represents the importance of the impact of the social construction of indigenous women as less than human mentioned in the introduction of this section. In yet another example of racism endangering Indigenous women, when two parents reported their daughter Jennifer missing in 2008, the investigating officers concluded, without providing evident reasoning that "she's [out drinking]... she'll be back". After the dismissive remarks, it was almost a month before the police decided to finally follow up with her whereabouts (National Inquiry, 2019a: 649–650). Lastly, similar excuses were provided to reason to why law enforcement in British Columbia failed to pursue an investigation which allowed a serial killer to murder forty-nine women, most of which were Indigenous, in Vancouver for more than a decade until the investigation was actually taken seriously and the killer was arrested and convicted (McClearn and Baum, 2015) and (Oppal, 2012) and (McGuire et al., 2022). As McGuire perfectly words it, "those women were mothers, sisters, and friends they were loved, and they are missed" (McGuire et al., 2022 p. 534). However, members of the justice system in Canada and the U.S are refusing to see indigenous women this way, and insteadapply stigmas and stereotypes to indigenous women which hinder their ability to efficiently conduct their jobs, which include protecting not only non-marginalized communities.

The structural racism of the criminal justice system includes the detainment of indigenous people as well. The overrepresentation of Indigenous peoples in Canada's federal correctional facilities is a well-documented reality in a lot of literature that discusses indigenous topics. While we could not get the statistics for Indigenous women in particular, studies report that in 2018–2019, Indigenous offenders represented 29% of the federally incarcerated population, comparable with 4.9% of the total Canadian population (Cameron et al., 2021). Also, compared to their non-Indigenous counterparts, Indigenous offenders are found more likely to be incarcerated at a younger age, denied parole and hence kept in custody longer, overrepresented in segregation and assigned the high-risk offender designation (Cameron et al., 2021). While these statistics do not include solely Indigenous women, we can imagine how the gendered impacts of being a woman adds on to this crisis, once again calling for attention to intersectionality.

The victimization against Indigenous women does not end with criminal justice system and extends to sexual violence within the medical field. Canada has a long and frightful history of reproductive coercion charged by long-standing eugenic principles (McKenzie et al., 2022). While Saskatchewan and Manitoba established sterilization acts that were combatted in the 1930s (Dyck, 2013), British Columbia and Alberta each had sexual sterilization legislation in effect not even a hundred years ago in the 20th century. Drafted sterilisation acts lasted from 1933 to 1973 in BC and from 1928 to 1972 in Alberta. Both Indigenous peoples and women were overrepresented among the cases presented to the Alberta Eugenics Board (Grekul et al., 2004 and (McKenzie et al., 2022). Research also proves that healthcare providers subjected Indigenous women in other provinces and territories to coercive sterilisation (Cohen & Baskett, 1978) and (Stote, 2012, 2015) and (McKenzie et al., 2022) despite such legislation not even existing.

Furthermore, Indigenous women in various locations in Canada (whether or not there were existing legislation acts) were subjected to unjust coercive practices related to abortion procedures and birth control. These practices were conducted through the ideas of colonial narratives that framed Indigenous women as both hypersexual and unqualified as mothers (Mckenzie et al., 2022).

However, reproductive coercion is not only a problem of the past. While Indigenous communities and media report anecdotal evidence of ongoing reproductive coercion to this day, according to McKenzie et al. analyses of contemporary Indigenous women's experiences is missing from current literature on reproductive coercion (McKenzie at al., 2022). Therefore, while western academia fails to report the ongoing methods of reproductive coercion in Canada, likely due to forms of discreteness in medical records, it is still a part of a vicious cycle of abuse indigenous women face from the medical field. Given that law enforcement does not take Indigenous safety in Canada seriously, this creates hindrances in being taken seriously when reporting the violence done against them by medical workers.

SOCIOECONOMIC IMPACT

In part by consequence of the various factors explored above, and deeply rooted within the historical and ongoing effects of colonialism, many Indigenous people face socioeconomic challenges. This section of the chapter includes mostly quantitative research of the ongoing economic injustice indigenous women face in Canada. To put these structural economic barriers into numbers, in 2016 census data proved that Indigenous total average income was $36,043, $47,981 for non-Indigenous people (Perreault, 2022). Due to these unequal pay gaps, GSS data also demonstrated that 22% of Indigenous people reported they have been unable to make payments, including scheduled bills and such, in a year preceding the survey. This is strikingly comparable to 10% of non-Indigenous people (Perreault, 2022). Furthermore, another study proved that 26% of Inuit, 24% of First Nations people and 11% of Métis live in a dwelling in need of major repairs, compared with 6.0% of non-Indigenous people (Statistics Canada, 2018). Lastly, 18% of

Indigenous people live in overcrowded living conditions, compared to only 8.5% of non-Indigenous people. The same study also highlighted that Indigenous people were much more likely than non-Indigenous people to experience food insecurity (Perreault, 2022).

Socioeconomic impacts are also reflected by the lack of access to adequate resources. Due to years of historical trauma resulting from colonialism and hence colonial related policies, as well as individual and systemic racism, many Indigenous women today face a multitude of deeply rooted social and economic challenges (Perreault, 2022). Many Indigenous communities and Indigenous people face limited and inequitable access or barriers (e.g., cultural barriers) to an extensive range of basic human services non-Indigenous people access effortlessly. These include health, education and employment services, which likely impacts their socioeconomic and health circumstances (Perreault, 2022). For example, GSS data shows that Indigenous people were more likely than non-Indigenous people to report that some services, such as shelters or transition homes, were not available in their area (17% versus 7.9%). Often, these obstacles are more frequent in rural or remote areas, where geography and population size may also present challenges in terms of services availability (Perreault, 2022).

However, in spite of these socioeconomic challenges, it is important to reflect on the benefits of Indigenous communities and culture that can alleviate the stress of these obstacles, and also look at some positive trends in the socioeconomic disadvantages. It is shown that Indigenous people benefit from levels of social factors that can mitigate the risk of violent victimisation (Perreault, 2022). For example, GSS data demonstrates that 27% of Indigenous people report a very strong sense of community belonging, this being compared with only 21% of their non-Indigenous counterparts. Additionally, 33% said they know most of the people in their neighbourhood (versus 15% on non-Indigenous people) , and 85% said their neighbourhood was a place where people help each other (Perreault, 2022). In addition, Indigenous people were more likely to report that their spiritual beliefs were very important to the way they live their life (35% compared to only 28% of non-

Indigenous people). These indicators may be reflective of strong social cohesion, which is known to be a protective factor from criminal victimisation (Perreault, 2022). Moreover, trends are showing that some socioeconomic gaps may be narrowing as of late. For example, the proportion of Indigenous people aged 20 to 24 with a high school diploma increased from 57% in 2006 to 70% in 2016, however a large gap still remains compared to non-Indigenous people from the same age group (91%) (Perreault,, 2022). This section is not to suggest there is still not a deep and structural problem with the socioeconomic challenges Indigenous women have to face. However, it is important to address the positive trends as well as the social life that may alleviate some of their stresses, signifying the importance of community in Indigenous life.

CONCLUSION

In this chapter, we have looked into multiple major structural factors that hinder Indigenous life for women. Within the three major structural factors we examined such as government legislations, the justice system including the medical field, and socioeconomic barriers include levels of even more obstacles that cause trouble in their daily lives. Of course, this is all by Western standards as fortunately their culture allows for their own community to rely and depend upon, which alleviates some of these strenuous impediments. However, attention to how being an Indigenous woman is critical of policy-makers to attack these structural forces as it still, and will always cause for unsafety in their lives if action is not taken immediately. The intersectionality of being a woman and Indigenous is important in the consideration of how current government policies and powers are working to make them feel neglected in Canada and the United States.

REFERENCES

Alfred T and Corntassel J (2005) Politics of identity – IX: Being indigenous: Resurgences against contemporary colonialism. Government and Opposition 40(4): 597–614.

Amnesty International (2008) Stolen sisters: A human rights response to discrimination and violence against indigenous women in Canada. Canadian Woman Studies 26(3/ 4): 105–121.

Balfour G (2008) Falling between the cracks of retributive and restorative justice: The victimization and punishment of aboriginal women. Feminist Criminology 3(2): 101–120.

Cameron, C., Khalifa, N., Bickle, A., Safdar, H., & Hassan, T. (2021). Psychiatry in the federal correctional system in canada. BJPsych International, 18(2), 42-46. doi:https://doi.org/10.1192/bji.2020.56

Cohen, J, & Baskett, TF (1978). Sterilization Patterns in a Northern Canadian Population. Canadian Journal of Public Health, 69(3), 222–224.

De Finney S (2017) Indigenous girls' resilience in settler states: Honouring body and land sovereignty. Agenda 31(2): 10–21.

Dyck, E. (2013). Facing eugenics: Reproduction, sterilization, and the politics of choice. University of Toronto Press.

Grekul, J., Krahn, A., & Odynak, D. (2004). Sterilizing the "feeble-minded": Eugenics in Alberta, Canada, 1929-1972. Journal of Historical Sociology, 17(4), 358–384. https:// doi.org/10.1111/j.1467-6443.2004.00237.x.

Indigenous Foundations. "Government Policy: The Indian Act". (2009). UBC. https://indigenousfoundations.arts.ubc.ca/home/

McGuire, M. M., & Murdoch, D. J. (2021). (in)-justice: An exploration of the dehumanization, victimization, criminalization, and over-incarceration of Indigenous Women in Canada. Punishment & Society, 24(4), 529–550. https://doi.org/10.1177/14624745211001685

McKenzie, H. A., Varcoe, C., Nason, D., McKenna, B., Lawford, K., Kelm, M.-E., Wajuntah, C. O., Gervais, L., Hoskins, J., Anaquod, J., Murdock, J., Murdock, R., Smith, K., Arkles, J., Acoose, S., & Arisman, K. (2022). Indigenous women's resistance of colonial policies,practices, and reproductive coercion. Qualitative Health Research, 32(7), 1031–1054. https://doi.org/10.1177/10497323221087526

McClearn M and Baum K (2015) Missing and murdered the taken: Who qualifies as a serial killer and more on the data behind the project. The Globe and Mail, 23 November. www.theglobeandmail.com/news/national/the-taken-wh o-qualifies-as-a-serial-killer-and-more-on-the-data-behind-the-project/arti cle27443307/

National Inquiry Into Missing and Murdered Indigenous Women and Girls (National Inquiry) (2019a) Reclaiming power and place: The final report of the National Inquiry into Missing and Murdered Indigenous women and Girls.

National Inquiry Into Missing and Murdered Indigenous Women and Girls (National Inquiry) (2019b) Reclaiming power and place: The final report of the National Inquiry into
Missing and Murdered Indigenous women and Girls. Volume 1b. Available at: www.mmiwg-ffada.ca/

Oppal WT (2012) Forsaken: The report of the Missing Women Commission of Inquiry ExecutiveSummary. Available at: www.missingwomeninquiry.ca/wp-content/uploads/2010/10/Forsaken-ES-web-RGB.pdf (accessed 6 August 2020).

Perreault, S. (2022). Victimization of first nations people, métis and inuit in canada.Juristat: Canadian Centre for Justice Statistics, , 1-72. http://libaccess.mcmaster.ca/login?url=https://www.proquest.com/scholarly-journals/victi mization-first-nations-people-métis-inuit/docview/2699769077/se-2

Razack S (1998) Looking white people in the eye: Gender, race, and culture in courtrooms and classrooms. Ontario: University of Toronto Press.

Statistics Canada. (2021). Housing conditions among First Nations people, Métis and Inuit in Canada from the 2021 Census. https://www12.statcan.gc.ca/census-recensement/2021/as-sa/ 98-200-X/2021007/98-200-X2021007-eng.cfm

Stote, K. (2012). The coercive sterilization of Aboriginal women in Canada. American Indian Culture and Research Journal, 36(3), 117–150. https://doi.org/10.17953/aicr.36.3. 7280728r6479j650.

Wesley M (2012) Marginalized: The aboriginal women's experience in federal corrections.Department of Public Safety and Emergency Preparedness. Available at:www.publicsafety.gc.ca/cnt/rsrcs/pblctns/mrgnlzd/mrgnlzd-eng.pdf (accessed 6 August 2020).

CHAPTER 8

RESPECTING INDIGENOUS PEOPLES AS A NON-INDIGENOUS PERSON: EXPLORING ALLYSHIP AND INTERSECTIONALITY FROM THE PERSPECTIVE OF AN ALLY

By Christina MacDonald

INTRODUCTION

Written from the perspective of a non-Indigenous person, this chapter aims to show respect for Indigenous Peoples by exploring resources that currently exist for non-Indigenous individuals to better understand what it means to be an ally. By delving into the concepts of allyship and intersectionality, this chapter aims to mobilise knowledge for those who want to learn more about being an ally but may not know where to start.

POSITIONALITY

Written from the perspective of a non-Indigenous person, this chapter does not claim to understand the trauma and unique life experiences of Indigenous Peoples. It is meant to be respectful towards Indigenous Peoples by exploring resources that currently exist for non-Indigenous individuals to better understand what it means to be an ally. By delving into the concepts of allyship and intersectionality, this chapter aims to mobilise knowledge for those who want to learn more about being an ally but may not know where to start.

LAYING THE FOUNDATION

Some important terms to understand in this chapter are allyship, intersectionality, cultural competence, cultural humility, and cultural safety. Within these concepts, social determinants of health, self-reflection, and self-reflexivity will also be discussed.

EXPLORING THE CONCEPT OF ALLYSHIP

An ally is not a label that can be given to anyone who expresses support for a group they do not belong to. Rather, practising allyship requires a commitment to constant learning, unlearning, and understanding that society has embedded systems that change how individuals live (The Anti-Oppression Network, n.d.).

It is important to be aware, however, that one's efforts are not performative. To be an ally means to actively evaluate one's position and understand that existing without fear of rejection and discrimination in certain societal contexts—such as attempting to receive health care services or looking for employment—is a sign of privilege (Thorne, 2022). To be performative is to want to show support without having the intention or desire to actively take part in change (Thorne, 2022). This is often seen on social media, where individuals will post at times of unrest, but will not actively seek out ways to help encourage change (Kalina, 2020). The message is not that one is expected to create change on their own, but it is about having the right intentions. To engage in allyship one must accept that allyship is not an empty term, but a constant and challenging process.

In her article entitled *The coin model of privilege and critical allyship: implications for health*, Nixon (2019) speaks to the concept of critical allyship. Nixon (2019) discusses how critical allyship is a process in which an individual must understand the societal inequities and privileges that exist. Practising critical allyship looks at the systems in place that perpetuate inequality and how actions can be taken to change the systems, not 'save' the people affected (Nixon, 2019). This concept will be explored in more depth in the next section about intersectionality as allyship and intersectionality are intertwined.

EXPLORING THE CONCEPT OF INTERSECTIONALITY

The term intersectionality was coined by Kimberlé W. Crenshaw, who wrote about it in the context of race and gender in her article *Demarginalizing the Intersection of Race and Sex: A Black Feminist Critique of Antidiscrimination Doctrine, Feminist Theory and Antiracist Politics* in 1989. Now, intersectionality is a lens that explores how different social structures discriminate against or oppress aspects of one's identity (Center for Intersectional Justice, n.d.). Factors such as race, disability, and gender and their social implications combine or intersect, in different ways, impacting one's experiences in society (Center for Intersectional Justice, n.d.). Intersectionality is linked with the concept of social determinants of health—factors that impact a person's health such as income, disability, race, food insecurity, housing, and many more (Raphael et al., 2020).

Intersectionality and the social determinants of health can be used to critically look at a variety of social systems that lead to oppression. An intersectional lens can be used when looking into respect and allyship in relation to Indigenous Peoples as it can help frame individual and collective experiences in a way that highlights privilege and oppression. Returning to *The coin model of privilege and critical allyship: implications for health, Nixon* (2019) provides a useful visual to understand intersectionality. In her article, a coin is used to visually represent inequality. It explains that the coin itself represents a system of inequality, meaning the aspects of society that create and perpetuate inequality (Nixon, 2019). The top of the coin represents privilege, highlighting the aspects of one's life that have brought them unearned advantages. The bottom of the coin represents the aspects of one's life that have brought unearned disadvantages (Nixon, 2019).

It is important to note that using an intersectional lens in this chapter is not meant to frame Indigeneity as an issue, but rather it is about understanding how colonisation and the historical marginalisation of Indigenous Peoples should not be ignored when learning how to be a better ally. When applying Indigeneity to the coin model, for example, it is not accurate to say that Indigeneity is a disadvantage, but rather that the social systems that are dominant in Western society disadvantage Indigenous Peoples because they do not include Indigenous ways of being and knowing. With that being said, an intersectional lens frequently overemphasises disadvantages rather than elevates the strengths of the individual or collective (Levac et al., 2018).

Levac et al. (2018) wrote that intersectionality is a lens that can start to explore the nuanced nature of human experience. In terms of Indigeneity within the context of Western society, modifying one's intersectional lens can help to highlight the history of colonisation and its impact on current social systems that perpetuate oppression (Levac et al., 2018). One variation of an intersectional lens that is discussed by Levac et al. (2018) is "Red intersectionality". In the words of Clark (2016, p. 51), "Red intersectionality recognizes the importance of local and traditional tribal/nation teachings, and the inter-generational connection between the past and the present". Although this quotation is pulled from an article in which Clark (2016, p. 51) writes about Red intersectionality in the context of "violence against Indigenous girls", the overall lens of incorporating Indigenous ways of knowing into the intersectional lens is important in the context of allyship. The phrase *Indigenous ways of knowing* acknowledges that Indigenous knowledge is vast, complex, and different between Indigenous communities, transcending the concept of social learning—learning from the people in one's life—for example, by learning from the land (Office of Indigenous Initiatives, n.d.).

UNDERSTANDING CULTURAL COMPETENCE, CULTURAL HUMILITY, AND CULTURAL SAFETY

Cultural competence, cultural humility, and cultural safety are terms used frequently in healthcare literature. These three terms are all important and, on the surface, may seem to have some overlap, but they are distinct concepts. To start, cultural competence focuses on the knowledge that allows a clinician to provide care that is respectful and aware of diverse client values and beliefs (Stubbe, 2020). It is important to highlight, however, that cultural competency has its limitations. The focus on knowledge implies that simply learning about another culture allows a clinician to be competent enough to engage with someone of the given culture (Stubbe, 2020). This fails to account for the client and their role in the client-clinician interaction; it also oversimplifies the idea of culture and how individual clients' identities within a given culture can be diverse (Beagan, 2018). Carey (2015) looks at cultural competence in relation to Indigenous studies in an Australian context and discusses how cultural competence over-emphasizes a dichotomy between Indigenous and non-Indigenous identities while also oversimplifying the idea of Indigenous identity, which in reality is extremely unique and diverse.

Beagan (2018) writes that cultural humility, on the other hand, goes a step further to an ongoing process in which a clinician interacts with their patient and honours their unique values and beliefs by constantly engaging in reflexivity and reflection (Beagan, 2018). This approach considers power and the imbalances there may be in a clinician-patient relationship (Beagan, 2018). To clarify, reflexivity and reflection are two separate terms that are both important to know and practice. Reflexivity is the active checking of one's assumptions and values that can bias their views (Cunliffe, 2016). Reflection, although likely more well-known, is different from reflexivity as it focuses on the analysis or 'reflection' of a given situation or learned information. Reflection can bring awareness to the meaning behind knowledge learned, but reflexivity allows one to delve deeper into the structures that have built and influenced the learner and those around them (Cunliffe, 2016).

In the context of Indigenous health, many systems in place create an inherent power imbalance. For example, Western healthcare systems do not effectively (if at all) integrate Indigenous ways of knowing into care. Not only that but there have also been several instances of racism and discrimination against Indigenous individuals in healthcare settings (Phillips-Beck et al., 2020), further highlighting the power imbalances in the systems that lead to oppression.

Cultural safety goes one step further and looks at power imbalances as embedded in systems (specifically the healthcare system in literature) (First Nations Health Authority, n.d.). It strives to address the impacts of these imbalances and the systems that are perpetuating inequalities to create a safe environment for those receiving care (First Nations Health Authority, n.d.). In addition to power imbalances and discrimination in healthcare systems, in an Indigenous context, cultural safety would also delve into colonization and the ever-existent impacts of colonialism on Indigenous health and the healthcare system (Baba, 2013).

RESOURCES THAT CAN ENCOURAGE COMPETENT, HUMBLE AND SAFE ALLYSHIP

Applying the concepts of cultural competence, cultural humility, and cultural safety to allyship can help to frame how one should approach being an ally to Indigenous Peoples. Mixing these concepts with allyship to create competent allyship, humble allyship and safe allyship (which are not official terms) helps to highlight that actively seeking out accurate information, engaging in continuous learning, and constantly engaging in reflective and reflexive practices on one's own position and the power they may hold. To be a learner means that one must consume information; to ensure accurate representation, resources that are written by or informed by Indigenous Peoples can be a great place to start. Some helpful resources that will be discussed in this chapter are the *Indigenous Ally Toolkit*, the *Decolonial Toolbox – Educational Pathway, KAIROS Blanket Exercise*, the *Anti-Racism, Cultural Safety & Humility Framework* and resources found on various university websites.

INDIGENOUS ALLY TOOLKIT

The *Indigenous Ally Toolkit* written by Swiftwolfe (2019) is an eight-page resource released by the Montreal Indigenous Community Network (the NETWORK). By encouraging readers to check their motivations, learn, and take action, the toolkit outlines important information for anyone who is trying to become an authentic ally. One aspect that is highlighted in this document that readers of this chapter should also take away is that it is important to learn information about Indigenous Peoples from Indigenous Peoples (Swiftwolfe, 2019). As much as this chapter aims to provide useful information, it strives to highlight Indigenous resources and demonstrate that part of allyship is knowing that there is a limit to what a non-Indigenous person can speak to and understand.

Moreover, understanding the power of language is brought up in the toolkit and suggestions have been implemented within this chapter. For example, this chapter uses the phrase "the Indigenous Peoples of what we now call Canada" instead of saying "Canada's Indigenous Peoples" because, as Swiftwolfe (2019) explains, one should not imply that Indigenous Peoples belong to Canada, nor should one use any possessive language when referring to Indigenous Peoples. In being more conscientious and meaningful with language, individuals striving to be genuine allies can actively demonstrate a commitment to challenging the power imbalances and inequalities in society.

It is also important to acknowledge that the term "Indigenous Peoples" in itself is a generalization. "[T]he Indigenous Peoples of what we now call Canada" maintain various beliefs, values, and ways of living depending on the community or communities they are a part of (Swiftwolfe, 2019). The Government of Canada (2022) acknowledges that Métis, First Nations and Inuit are distinct Peoples, but this does not even begin to explore the multitude of Indigenous cultures, languages, and communities (Government of Canada, 2022). Swiftwolfe (2019) speaks to how "Indigenous culture" is not specific enough of a term because it does not capture the nuanced complexity of various Indigenous identities.

Overall, the toolkit is a useful resource for allies or individuals who are striving to practice authentic allyship.

DECOLONIAL TOOLBOX – EDUCATIONAL PATHWAY

The *Decolonial Toolbox* is another resource on the NETWORK's website that was made as a way to provide the general public with information about Indigenous experiences, by Indigenous Peoples (Sioui et al., 2022a). The toolbox has been created over several years with the efforts of the Office of Community Engagement at Concordia University, Mikana, an Indigenous non-profit organization, and the NETWORK (Sioui et al., 2022a). The resource is currently split into three different downloadable documents: *Decolonial Toolbox – Educational Pathway, Level 1: Introduction to Indigenous Realities, and Level 2: Colonial Strategies*. The initial introductory document mentions that it is a five-level path, indicating that there will likely be three more documents to be released.

The first document is a four-page introduction to the resource, providing background on why it was created. It highlights to readers that the goal is to increase one's understanding of decolonization to provide tools for individuals to start altering and adopting mindsets that help to encourage change (Sioui et al., 2022a). The second document, *Level 1: Introduction to Indigenous Realities*, is a three-page document that focuses on important terminology and changing one's understanding of Indigenous experiences by providing resources that highlight Indigenous stories from Indigenous perspectives, rather than the widely perpetuated colonial perspectives on Indigenous lives (Sioui et al., 2022b). The third document, *Level 2: Colonial Strategies*, is a seven-page document that delves deeper into colonialism and the history of colonialism on Indigenous Peoples (Sioui et al., 2022c). It educates readers about historical colonial events that caused significant trauma and displacement. For example, the Indian Act and the creation and enforcement of residential schools. This chapter will not delve into these topics, but they are all important to learn about to increase one's knowledge and ability to be a genuine ally.

Both the Level 1 and Level 2 documents are filled with links to videos, articles, and otherresources related to the information being provided. The toolbox is a comprehensive resource that can be utilised by individuals aiming to work on Indigenous allyship because it is directly written for the public with an understanding that they may not have exposure to Indigenous ways of knowing nor to resources that do not inherently perpetuate colonial values.

KAIROS BLANKET EXERCISE

KAIROS Blanket Exercise may not be accessible to all, as there is a cost, but if the opportunity arises, this could be a useful learning opportunity. It should be noted, however, that the costs are flexible in an effort to make the workshop more accessible (KAIROS Blanket Exercise Community, n.d.a). There is also a newer virtual version of the workshop that was created due to the COVID-19 pandemic bringing forward the utility of virtual gathering spaces (KAIROS Blanket Exercise Community, n.d.b).

As Lakehead University (n.d.) describes it, "KAIROS Blanket Exercise is an experiential workshop that explores the nation-to-nation relationship between Indigenous and non-Indigenous peoples in Canada". Participants are able to engage in active learning as they learn about how the land (represented with blankets) was impacted by colonisation from the perspectives of First Nations, Inuit, And Métis Peoples (Lakehead University, n.d.).

Thinking about the implications of this workshop on allyship, non-Indigenous individuals can use this learning opportunity to engage in reflexive practices and build their cultural humility. Although allyship involves action, taking opportunities to learn and challenge one's current understanding of Indigenous Peoples is an important step in the process.

ANTI-RACISM, CULTURAL SAFETY & HUMILITY FRAMEWORK

The *Anti-Racism, Cultural Safety & Humility Framework* is a ten-page document based out of British Columbia and a collaborative work from the First Nations Health Authority (FNHA), First Nations Health Council (FNHC), and First Nations Health Directors Association (FNHDA) (2021). The document encourages action to eliminate discrimination and racism against First Nations. Although this document is not specific to allyship at an individual level, it provides useful information about efforts being made to create change in the healthcare system that may promote one's learning and knowledge of current system inequalities (FNHA, FNHC, & FNHDA, 2021). For individuals, it can be helpful to become more familiar with the higher-level systems and ongoing attempts to create change. In knowing what organisations and groups are setting standards for care and making the effort to implement culturally safe systems, one can use them as resources to further their knowledge. For example, this framework document provides useful definitions and highlights system gaps that need to be actively addressed.

VARIOUS UNIVERSITY WEBSITES

Whether or not one is affiliated with a university, university websites often have pages with information, resources, articles and links to other sites to enhance one's knowledge about Indigenous Peoples and their various cultures, traditions and beliefs. They often have several resources created or informed by Indigenous Peoples. Moreover, several universities will have departments or offices for Indigenous studies, services, learning, health, and more. For example, McMaster University in Hamilton, Ontario has an Indigenous Student Services website, the University of Manitoba in Winnipeg, Manitoba has an Indigenous Student Centre website, and Queen's University in Kingston, Ontario has an Office of Indigenous Initiatives website.

University sites may include land acknowledgments to honour the territories on which they are situated, so if one would like to learn more about specific territories and the history of the colonisation of the land, there are often resources specific to the universities' locations.

If one does not know where to start, one can take advantage of the resources the universities have to offer by searching the university name on the Internet and including the word 'Indigenous' or 'Indigenous services' in the search. This section is referring to Canadian universities specifically but can likely be applied to universities in other countries as well.

IT IS NEVER TOO LATE TO START LEARNING

Allyship is challenging and lifelong. Returning to the concept of cultural humility, being an ally requires a commitment to being reflexive and continually seeking out new information to better oneself. Thinking about the development of one's intersectional lens, participating in workshops, reading Indigenous-written resources, and questioning one's own biases and assumptions can encourage more authentic allyship.

REFERENCES

Baba, L. (2013). Cultural safety in First Nations, Inuit and Métis public health: Environmental scan of cultural competency and safety in education, training and health services. Prince George, BC: National Collaborating Centre for Aboriginal Health. https://www.ccnsa-nccah.ca/docs/emerging/RPT-CulturalSafetyPublicHealth-BabaEN.pdf

Beagan, B. L. (2018). A critique of cultural competence: Assumptions, limitations, and alternatives. In C. Frisby & W. O'Donohue (Eds.), Cultural Competence in Applied Psychology. Springer, Cham. https://doi.org/10.1007/978-3-319-78997-2_6

Carey, M. (2015). The limits of cultural competence: an Indigenous Studies perspective. Higher Education Research & Development, 34(5), 828–840. https://doi.org/10.1080/07294360.2015.1011097

Center for Intersectional Justice. (n.d.). What is intersectionality. https://www.intersectionaljustice.org/what-is-intersectionality

Clark, N. (2016). Red intersectionality and violence-informed witnessing praxis with Indigenous girls. Girlhood Studies, 9(2), 46–64. https://doi.org/10.3167/ghs.2016.090205

Crenshaw, K. (1989). Demarginalizing the intersection of race and sex: A Black feminist critique of antidiscrimination doctrine, feminist theory and antiracist politics. University of Chicago Legal Forum, 140, 139–167.

Cunliffe, A. (2016), Republication of "on becoming a critically reflexive practitioner". Journal of Management Education, 40(6), 747–768. https://doi.org/10.1177/1052562916674465

First Nations Health Authority, First Nations Health Council, & First Nations Health Director's Association. (2021, April 2022). Anti-Racism, Cultural Safety

& Humility Framework. https://www.fnha.ca/Documents/FNHA-FNHC-FNHDA-Anti-Racism-Cultural-Safetyand-Humility-Framework.pdf

First Nations Health Authority. (n.d.). Creating a climate for change. https://www.fnha.ca/Documents/FNHA-Creating-a-Climate-For-Change-CulturalHumility-Resource-Booklet.pdf

Government of Canada. (2022, June 13). Learn more about First Nations, Inuit, and Métis Peoples across Canada. https://www.rcaanc-cirnac.gc.ca/eng/1621447127773/1621447157184

KAIROS Blanket Exercise Community. (n.d.a). Frequently asked questions. https://www.kairosblanketexercise.org/frequently-asked-questions/#cost

KAIROS Blanket Exercise Community. (n.d.b). KAIROS Blanket Exercise. https://www.kairosblanketexercise.org/

Kalina, P. (2020). Performative allyship. Technicum Social Sciences Journal, 11, 478–481.

Lakehead University. (n.d.). University community KAIROS Blanket Exercise. https://www.lakeheadu.ca/indigenous/recruitment-outreach/KAIROS

Levac, L., McMurtry, L., Stienstra, D., Baikie, G., Hanson, C., & Mucina, D. (2018). Learning across Indigenous and Western knowledge systems and intersectionality: Reconcilingsocial science research approaches. University of Guelph. https://doi.org/10.13140/RG.2.2.19973.65763

Office of Indigenous Initiatives. (n.d.) Ways of knowing. Queen's University. https://www.queensu.ca/indigenous/ways-knowing/about

Phillips-Beck, W., Eni, R., Lavoie, J. G., Avery Kinew, K., Kyoon Achan, G., & Katz, A. (2020). Confronting racism within the Canadian healthcare system: Systemic exclusion of First Nations from quality and consistent care. International Journal of Environmental Research and Public Health, 17(22), 8343. https://doi.org/10.3390/ijerph17228343

Nixon, S. A. (2019). The coin model of privilege and critical allyship: implications for health. BMC Public Health, 19(1637). https://doi.org/10.1186/s12889-019-7884-9

Raphael, D., Bryant, T., Mikkonen, J., & Raphael, A. (2022). Social determinants of health: The Canadian fact (2nd ed). Oshawa: Ontario Tech University Faculty of Health Sciences and Toronto: York University School of Health Policy and Management. https://thecanadianfacts.org/The_Canadian_Facts-2nd_ed.pdf

Sioui, A., Moniz, A., Cohen-Bucher, E., & Sioui, G. (2022a). Decolonial toolbox: Educational pathway. https://reseaumtlnetwork.com/wp- content/uploads/2022/06/EN_Educational_Pathway_Final_june2022_V2_compressed-1-4.pdf

Sioui, A., Moniz, A., Cohen-Bucher, E., & Sioui, G. (2022b). Level 1: Introduction to Indigenous realities. https://reseaumtlnetwork.com/wpcontent/uploads/2022/06/EN_Educational_Pathway_Final_june2022_V2_compressed-5-7.pdf

Sioui, A., Moniz, A., Cohen-Bucher, E., & Sioui, G. (2022c). Level 2: Colonial strategies. https://reseaumtlnetwork.com/wpcontent/uploads/2022/06/EN_Educational_Pathway_Final_june2022_V2_compressed-8- 14.pdf

Stubbe, D. E. (2020). Practicing cultural competence and cultural humility in the care of diverse patients. Focus, 18(1), 49–51. https://doi.org/10.1176/appi.focus.20190041

Swiftwolfe, D. (2019, March). Indigenous ally toolkit. Montreal Urban Aboriginal Community Strategy Network. https://reseaumtlnetwork.com/wpcontent/uploads/2019/04/Ally_March.pdf

The Anti-Oppression Network. (n.d.). Allyship. https://theantioppressionnetwork.com/allyship/

Thorne, S. (2022). Moving beyond performative allyship. Nursing Inquiry, 29(1), e12483. https://doi-org.libaccess.lib.mcmaster.ca/10.1111/nin.12483

CHAPTER 9

EXPLORING THE OVERREPRESENTATION OF INDIGENOUS CHILDREN IN FOSTER CARE

By Rida Khan

SUMMARY

The Canadian Child Welfare system has clear overrepresentation of Indigenous youth due to the discriminatory biases shown by child welfare workers. This as an extension of residential school systems and can lead to detrimental and differential impact on Indigenous youth. Efforts towards reconciliation must be implemented.

INTRODUCTION

Foster care, or out-of-home care, is the removal of a child or youth from their family and placement into a government-directed substitute family environment in the home of foster parents (Pinderhughes & Fermin, 2011). In Canada, 26,680 children from birth to age 14 are in foster care as of 2021 (Statistics Canada, 2021). However, of these children, there is a large overrepresentation of Indigenous children in out-of-home care. This overrepresentation can be rooted in systemic discrimination and the intergenerational effects of residential schools. This leads to long-term consequences for Indigenous children as they struggle with mental health, loss of social support and loss of cultural identity. The following chapter will explore the causes and consequences of the current child welfare crisis faced by Indigenous children and the policies that have been made to tackle these systemic issues.

THE CURRENT OVERREPRESENTATION OF INDIGENOUS CHILDREN IN CANADA'S CHILD WELFARE SYSTEM

According to the 2021 census conducted by Statistics Canada, 7.7% of all children in Canada that are under 14 are Indigenous (Government of Canada, 2020). In comparison, 53.8% of children in foster care are indigenous (Government of Canada, 2020). Overall, this represents the disparity and overrepresentation that Is currently present for Indigenous children. This is not the first instance where Indigenous children have had higher rates of separation from their families. The Canadian government has had a long history of separating Indigenous children from their families through residential schools. This over-representation of indigenous children is indicative of systemic racial discrimination that these children face and contributes to negative outcomes seen amongst Indigenous children who grew up within Canadian child welfare systems. As indigenous populations continue to grow, it becomes increasingly important to recognize this overrepresentation and integrate social policies to remove these disparities.

DISCRIMINATORY BIAS FACED BY INDIGENOUS FAMILIES

The overrepresentation of indigenous children in foster care is due to discriminatory bias in policies and decision-making of the Canadian government. Firstly, this discriminatory bias begins with the elementary schools and medical centers where indigenous families interact with the public sector. For instance, studies from the United States demonstrate evidence of schools and medical staff over-reporting racialized families to child welfare authorities based on maltreatment and neglect, despite controlling for the likelihood of abusive injury (Font et al., 2012). This can create a larger impact on Indigenous families as false reports of maltreatment result in greater proportions of indigenous children being admitted into foster care despite living in healthy atmospheres. These studies can be reflected in Canadian populations, since a study conducted in 2008 found that one out of seven First Nations children in areas included in the First Nations Component of the Canadian Incidence Study of Reported Child Abuse and Neglect was subject to a new child welfare investigation (Caldwell & Sinha, 2020).

In the same year, child maltreatment-related investigation involving First Nations children was 4.2 times greater than for non-Aboriginal children (Caldwell & Sinha, 2020). This may indicate that the true reason for the overrepresentation of indigenous youth in foster care is due to preconceived racial biases that result in false identification of maltreatment or abuse. Other statistics show that investigation for neglect are 8.5 times higher in Indigenous children than non-indigenous, exposure to intimate partner violence is 4.2 times higher, and emotional maltreatment is 3.1 times higher (First Nations Canadian Incidence Study, 2019). Despite this, physical harm was only documented 4$ of the substantiated maltreatment investigation involving First Nations children (First Nations Canadian Incidence Study, 2019). Out of home care became 17.1 times higher for indigenous children than non-indigenous children (First Nations Canadian Incidence Study, 2019). Therefore, discriminatory bias is evident in the reports and investigations by the Canadian protective services towards Indigenous families, resulting in greater rates of child separation. These disparities in reported investigations of Indigenous families can be indicative of discriminatory biases that influence decision and policymaking in their community services such as healthcare, schools, and daycare centers. These higher rates of investigation for child maltreatment, intimate partner violence and failure to provide care may be due to higher rates of visibility bias, which is the greater exposure of First Nation people to reporters due to structural issues such as poverty and violence.

This practice of discriminatory bias resulting in greater rates of Indigenous youth being put into child welfare is indicative of the colonialism that is forced upon them. The racist ideologies of governments had forced the development of the residential school system, where children were removed from their homes and separated from their families to eradicate their culture and assimilate children into the colonial norms. Similarly, the overrepresentation of Indigenous children has a similar impact to parental separation and may contribute to the effort to eradicate Indigenous culture and create inequity. For instance, in the 1950s, over 20,000 Indigenous children were removed from their homes and put into the child welfare system at a time known as the

"Sixties Scoop". This was to eradicate an Indigenous culture, their familial and community support, and their identity. As a result, the overrepresentation of Indigenous children in welfare is a malicious yet subtle extension of the impacts of residential schools.

INTERGENERATIONAL EFFECTS OF RESIDENTIAL SCHOOLS

Indigenous communities have historically faced years of oppression and familial separation through residential schools. Residential school systems were introduced by colonial settlers intended to eradicate language, cultural traditions and spiritual beliefs of Indigenous children (Wilk et al., 2017). More than 150,000 indigenous children were stolen from their families and assimilated into Canadian society between the 1870s and the mid-1990s (Wilk et al., 2017). Although many residential schools have since shut down, the intergenerational impacts of residential schools continue to impact indigenous communities to this day (Wilk et al., 2017). The increased removal of children from their homes into child welfare is a continuation of Canada's colonial history with Indigenous communities.

Overrepresentation of indigenous children in child welfare is related to intergenerational trauma from residential schools. Studies in British Columbia found that Indigenous children who had either a parent or grandparent that attended residential school are more than two times more likely to be in government care (Barker et al., 2019). Indigenous children of survivors of residential school systems experience increased negative physical and mental health issues, including higher rates of suicidal ideation and attempts compared to individuals without a parent that attended residential school (Bombay et al., 2014). The highest reasons for children being reported to child welfare services is due to parental substance abuse, neglect, intimate partner violence, food insecurity, and poverty (Bombay et al., 2014). These factors are also characterized by the collective generational trauma and impacts of residential school systems which lead to increased risk for negative health and social outcomes for Indigenous youth and parents (Bombay et al., 2014).

Exposure to the Indigenous residential school systems also contributes to increased representation of Indigenous children due to the systemic conditions it left Indigenous adult survivors. Residential schools resulted in Indigenous children, and today's parents, to be disconnected from cultural and loving child rearing practises, their own community elders, parental role models, cultures and identities (Bombay et al., 2020). Consequences also included medical and psychosomatic conditions, mental health conditions and post-traumatic stress disorder and dysregulated emotional well-being (Wilk et al., 2017). Despite the profound effects of residential schools, survivors were provided with no financial resources to address these issues or to support their new families. Children of survivors were therefore more vulnerable to poverty, food insecurity, abuse and neglect which can be related to negative health outcomes or school success (Bombay et al., 2020). Rather than providing reconciliation and support to these families to allow them to heal from trauma, policies favoured the removal of children from their homes (de Leeuw et al., 2009).

THE DETRIMENTAL IMPACT OF CHILD WELFARE ON INDIGENOUS CHILDREN

The higher rates of indigenous children being taken into child welfare and separated from their families are associated with many negative and long-term mental health consequences faced by these children. According to study by the National Youth Homelessness Survey, it was found that children with an involvement of child protection services show higher rates of chronic homelessness, at 35.6%, compared to those who did not, at 26.9%. Additionally, 31.5% of indigenous youth in general already face homelessness in Canada (Gaetz, n.d.). They also face lower rates of post-secondary education as while 12% of the student population in B.C. is Indigenous, about 67% of youth in care identify as Indigenous Indigenous children and youth in government care experience poorer education outcomes than students in the general population. For example, the 2016-17 six-year public school completion rate for Indigenous students in government care in B.C. was 44.1%, while the public-school completion rate for all students in B.C. was 83.7% (Government of Canada, 2019). These children face low levels of post-secondary education, low income, high employment, and increased prevalence of chronic disease (Ontario Human Rights Council, n.d.). Compared to the general population, they are also more likely to be involved in the criminal justice system. These repercussions are all related to long-term resolved trauma, permanent mistrust of institutions, and deep feelings of cultural disconnection and loss of identity due to a loss of cultural identity. There is also a loss of resources to help those children who are suffering with mental health and struggles such as addiction and poverty. (Ontario Human Rights Commission, n.d.)

Although there is limited data on child welfare in Canada, there is available studied that strongly link child welfare data in Canada to distress among indigenous youth. It was found from the Aboriginal Peoples Survey in 2006 that Metis adults who had been placed into child welfare as children are more likely to have has more recent depressive episodes and lifetime suicide ideation than those who has never been in care (Kidd et al., 2019). Another study in British Columbia also found that children who had been placed in foster care homes were more likely to experience self-harm, suicide ideation and attempts, drug overdose, homelessness, or risky behaviours (Clarkson, 2015). Due to the long-term mental health effects that individuals who are put into child welfare endure, this system of overrepresentation might contribute to the long-lasting intergeneration trauma and inequities experienced by Indigenous children, similar to the residential school system.

The "Sixties Scoop" was a period in the 1950s in which child welfare authorities removed thousands of Indigenous children from their families and communities in great numbers (Allen et al., 2020). These children were send to be fostered or adopted in mostly non-Indigenous families (Allen et al., 2020). Survivors of the "Sixties Scoop" had drastically exasperated mental illness and addiction experiences, which is now referred to as "soul wound" by indigenous community members (Allen et al., 2020). A survivor from the Sixties Scoop, Christine Miskonoodinkwe Smith, shared her experience in foster care and said, "I was adopted with my biological sister. We were physically and emotionally abused. From a very young age, I was constantly being told I was a little bitch.

That I wasn't going to amount to anything. That I was stupid. I went into foster care at age 10. It wasn't until my third foster home that I realized that the people taking me in actually cared. I experienced trauma and rejection and was in and out of the hospital for much of my 20s" (Marwaha, 2020). This real life experience goes to show the true impact of separating indigenous children from their families leading to life-long mistrust of healthcare systems, detrimental mental health consequences and trauma.

During the "Sixties Scoop", many children were placed in distant communities and exported to other provinces or across the US border to the homes of middle-class white families (Kulusic, 2005). Placement with non-Indigenous communities led to a destruction of cultural knowledge and cultural continuity, as children were not placed in culturally appropriate foster homes, but rather distant and westernized homes and their cultural needs were ignored (Alston-O'Connor, 2010). Cultural separation has been shown to be a social determinant of health (Kim, 2019). Loss of culture can lead to major risk for mental disorders and can cause dysregulation of brain function later in life (Kim, 2019). Additionally, children experience feelings of cultural shame and disconnection which is associated with mental health problems, homelessness and incarceration (McQuaid et al., 2022). Therefore, cultural separation due to child welfare results in detriments to child health. Ultimately, the overrepresentation of Indigenous youth in child welfare has been shown to have long-term negative consequences on their well-being.

PATHWAY TOWARDS TACKLING A FLAWED SYSTEM

An Act Respecting First nations, Inuit and Metis Children

The current crisis of Indigenous children in child welfare systems is becoming recognized by policymakers who are developing interventions to improve Indigenous children's well-being. The National Truth and Reconciliation Commission of Canada works towards calling attention to the damage that was induced by government policies and practises upon Indigenous communities (Government of Canada, 2018) The National Truth and

Reconciliation Act has placed the crisis of child welfare at a top priority, calling on the government to ensure equitable funding for Indigenous child welfare agencies and recognizing that Indigenous communities should be involved in decision-making (National Collaborating Center for Aboriginal Health, 2017). In 2019, the federal government co-developed a bill with Indigenous partners called the "Act respecting First Nations, Inuit and Métis children, youth and families", aiming to reform child welfare and improve outcomes for Indigenous children (Government of Canada, 2020). This includes principles of "cultural continuity" and "substantive equality" of child and family service provision as being essential to the child's well-being (Government of Canada, 2020). They also seek to recognize the rights of Indigenous governing bodies and communities in decision-making for Indigenous children (Government of Canada, 2020).

As a step towards ensuring the most beneficial decisions are made for the child, in cases of familial separation and child relocation from their homes, the act has allows First Nations, Inuit and Metis peoples to exercise jurisdiction over and child and family services (Government of Canada, 2018a). As a result, Indigenous community leaders were able to develop their own child and family services models, systems and laws that are rooted in true indigenous values, languages and cultures (Government of Canada, 2018b). This allowed children to stay connected and involved in their own Indigenous culture and prioritize the promotion of their culture despite relocation to non-indigenous homes.

Increasing Research on Indigenous Children in Child Welfare

The Public Health Agency of Canada has also collaborated to work on the "Pan-Northern Data Project" to increase available data about children in care and reasons for apprehension (Government of Canada, 2018). This creates the opportunity to develop interventions to combat harmful systemic discriminatory bias against Indigenous families and ensure the opportunity for Indigenous communities to tell their stories. Additional funding of over $542 million over 5 years was allocated by the Government of Canada to support the implementation of this act (Government of Canada, 2018). Ultimately, policymakers are recognizing and tackling the child welfare crisis while collaborating with Indigenous community partners.

Making Institutions Safer for Indigenous Children

On a smaller scale as well, reconciliation must also take place at a community level to eradicate the biases and discrimination faced by Indigenous families. For instance, schools and health care facilities must focus on re-establishing trust with Indigenous leaders and families (Milne & Wotherspoon, 2020). Although schools should be a supportive, safe and secure environment for indigenous children to socialize, learn and find success, institutions like these can produce stress and anxiety which repels Indigenous children from going to school or interacting with educators (Milne & Wotherspoon, 2020). As previously mentioned, most reports for maltreatment investigation start at these institutions where Indigenous families interact with their children's teachers and may face stereotype biases (Ma et al., 2019). As a result, it is important for provincial and territorial education ministries to prioritize cultural competence and embed Indigenous cultural norms and knowledge into teacher's responsibilities and teaching education (Milne & Wotherspoon, 2020).

Ontario's Child Welfare Re-Design Strategy

It has been shown and discussed that community connection, sense of belonging and identity have become increasingly important in maintaining the well-being of Indigenous children. In response, Ontario's Child Welfare Re-Design Strategy has been implemented in hopes to strengthening familial ties and communities for children in foster care by providing culturally appropriate resources (Quinn, 2022). This framework was released on July 29, 2020 and was designed with input from youth, families, caregivers, and Indigenous community partners (Ministry of Children, Community and Social Services, 2020). The design will help strengthen families ties and improve quality of residential care provided to children and youth by training caregivers (Ministry of Children, Community and Social Services, 2020). Additionally, the design will introduce strengthened youth supports with a focus on education and employment to improve outcomes of youth while reducing poverty rates (Ministry of Children, Community and Social Services, 2020). Finally, this design will improve the adoption experience for children, youth and prospective parents and create a child welfare system that is more financially sustainable (Ministry of Children, Community and Social Services, 2020).

Ultimately, although steps have been made to try to reduce the number of Indigenous children in foster care, the fraction of Indigenous children in child welfare is still increasing. Indigenous children in child welfare increased from 52.2% in 2016 to 53.8% in 2021 (Government of Canada, 2016). Therefore, the overrepresentation problem is still present and should be prioritized in order to fulfil reconciliation with Indigenous communities.

CONCLUSION

Indigenous communities faced years of intergenerational trauma due to the residential school system however, inequity continues to be embodied under the disguise of child welfare. The overrepresentation of children in child welfare is associated with the discriminatory bias of decision-makers and the long-lasting effects of intergenerational trauma amongst families. This results in negative consequences for the mental health and cultural identity of Indigenous youth, resulting in a response from the Government which began to create policies to alleviate the child welfare crisis. Governments must continue to implement these policies to create long overdue equity and justice for Indigenous communities.

REFERENCES

Allen, L., Hatala, A., Ijaz, S., Courchene, E. D., & Bushie, E. B. (2020). Indigenous-led health care partnerships in Canada. CMAJ : Canadian Medical Association Journal, 192(9), E208–E216. https://doi.org/10.1503/cmaj.190728

Alston-O'Connor, E. (2010). The Sixties Scoop: Implications for Social Workers and Social Work Education. Critical Social Work, 11(1), Article 1. https://doi.org/10.22329/csw.v11i1.5816

Barker, B., Sedgemore, K., Tourangeau, M., Lagimodiere, L., Milloy, J., Dong, H., Hayashi, K., Shoveller, J., Kerr, T., & DeBeck, K. (2019). Intergenerational Trauma: The Relationship Between Residential Schools and the Child Welfare System Among Young People Who Use Drugs in Vancouver, Canada. Journal of Adolescent Health, 65(2), 248–254. https://doi.org/10.1016/j.jadohealth.2019.01.022

Bombay, A., McQuaid, R., Young, J., Sinha, V., Currie, V., Anisman, H., & Matheson, K. (2020). Familial Attendance at Indian Residential School and Subsequent Involvement in the Child Welfare System Among Indigenous Adults Born During the Sixties Scoop Era. First Peoples Child & Family Review: An Interdisciplinary Journal Honouring the Voices, Perspectives, and Knowledges of First Peoples, 15(1), 62–79. https://doi.org/10.7202/1068363ar

Clarkson, A. F., Christian, W. M., Pearce, M. E., Jongbloed, K. A., Caron, N. R., Teegee, M. P., Moniruzzaman, A., Schechter, M. T., Spittal, P. M., & For the Cedar Project Partnership. (2015). The Cedar Project: Negative health outcomes associated with involvement in the child welfare system among young Indigenous people who use injection and non-injection drugs in two Canadian cities. Canadian Journal of Public Health, 106(5), e265–e270. https://doi.org/10.17269/cjph.106.5026

de Leeuw, S., Greenwood, M., & Cameron, E. (2009). Deviant Constructions: How Governments Preserve Colonial Narratives of Addictions and Poor Mental Health to Intervene into the Lives of Indigenous Children and Families in Canada. International Journal of Mental Health and Addiction, 8, 282–295. https://doi.org/10.1007/s11469-009-9225-1

Government of Canada. (2018a, April 23). Child welfare [Guide]. https://www.rcaanc-cirnac.gc.ca/eng/1524494379788/1557513026413

Government of Canada. (2018, November 2). Reducing the number of Indigenous children in care [Fact sheet]. https://www.sac-isc.gc.ca/eng/1541187352297/1541187392851

Government of Canada, S. C. (2016, April 13). Living arrangements of Aboriginal children aged 14 and under. https://www150.statcan.gc.ca/n1/pub/75 006-x/2016001/article/14547-eng.htm

Kidd, S. A., Thistle, J., Beaulieu, T., O'Grady, B., & Gaetz, S. (2019). A national study of Indigenous youth homelessness in Canada. Public Health, 176, 163–171. https://doi.org/10.1016/j.puhe.2018.06.012

Kim, P. J. (2019). Social Determinants of Health Inequities in Indigenous Canadians Through a Life Course Approach to Colonialism and the Residential School System. Health Equity, 3(1), 378–381. https://doi.org/10.1089/heq.2019.0041

Ma, J., Fallon, B., & Richard, K. (2019). The overrepresentation of First Nations children and families involved with child welfare: Findings from the Ontario incidence study of reported child abuse and neglect 2013. Child Abuse & Neglect, 90, 52–65. https://doi.org/10.1016/j.chiabu.2019.01.022

Marwaha, S. (2020). Christine Miskonoodinkwe Smith. CMAJ : Canadian Medical Association Journal, 192(19), E526. https://doi.org/10.1503/cmaj.200620

McQuaid, R. J., Schwartz, F. D., Blackstock, C., Matheson, K., Anisman, H., & Bombay, A. (2022). Parent-Child Separations and Mental Health among First Nations and Métis Peoples in Canada: Links to Intergenerational Residential School Attendance. International Journal of Environmental Research and Public Health, 19(11), Article 11. https://doi.org/10.3390/ijerph19116877

Milne, E., & Wotherspoon, T. (2020). Schools as "Really Dangerous Places" for Indigenous Children and Youth: Schools, Child Welfare, and Contemporary Challenges to Reconciliation. Canadian Review of Sociology/Revue Canadienne de Sociologie, 57(1), 34–52. https://doi.org/10.1111/cars.12267

Ministry of Children, Community and Social Services. (2020, July 29). Child welfare redesign strategy. Ontario.Ca. https://www.children.gov.on.ca/htdocs/English/professionals/childwelfare/redesign-strategy.aspx National Collaborating Center for Aboriginal Health. (2017). Indigenous Children and the Child Welfare System in Canada. National Collaborating Center for Aboriginal Health. https://www.nccih.ca/docs/health/FS-ChildWelfareCanada-EN

Pinderhughes, E. E., & Fermin, L. L. (2011). Foster Care. In B. B. Brown & M. J. Prinstein (Eds.), Encyclopedia of Adolescence (pp. 95–98). Academic Press. https://doi.org/10.1016/B978-0-12-373951-3.00054-5

Quinn, A. L. (2022). Experiences and well-being among Indigenous former youth in care within Canada. Child Abuse & Neglect, 123, 105395. https://doi.org/10.1016/j.chiabu.2021.105395

Wilk, P., Maltby, A., & Cooke, M. (2017). Residential schools and the effects on Indigenous health and well-being in Canada—A scoping review. Public Health Reviews, 38, 8. https://doi.org/10.1186/s40985-017-0055-6

CHAPTER 10

THE EDUCATION GAP IN INDIGENOUS COMMUNITIES

By Razan Ahmed

INTRODUCTION

This country has a concerning Indigenous Education Gap—a disparity in educational achievement between Indigenous and non-Indigenous people. The Indigenous Education Gap is widening and rising quickly across Canada. Bridging the education gap is thus a critical component of any plan for enhancing the prosperity, health, and well-being of Canada's indigenous population, as well as eliminating marginalisation.

Education is one of the many concerns that Indigenous people in Canada must tackle. The acts of previous Canadian administrations, both implicit and explicit, have resulted in a considerable educational disparity between Indigenous and non-Indigenous pupils. The western system of education is inherently exclusive, and its fundamental educational process is based on privilege. Resolving the enormous and ongoing inequalities in student educational learning results must be based on Indigenous notions of education, rather than a standard western/colonial approach.

ELEMENTARY/HIGH SCHOOL EDUCATION

Indigenous education is severely underfunded, particularly on reserves. The issue is that federal funds are used to finance First Nations schools, while provincial funds are used to fund other schools. Schools on reserves are predicted to receive at least 30% less money than regular schools (Derenisky, 2020). First Nations schools receive far less funding per student than other schools. This indicates that Indigenous children receive considerably less financing for their schooling if they opt to live on their ancestral reserve land with their families. This makes it more difficult for these schools to deliver the same level of education. It also makes it difficult for them to give extra assistance to students who must leave their reservation to attend high school in a city. Because of their distant location and limited size, schools on reserves already have greater expenditures, and having less financing creates an even wider imbalance. (Derenisky, 2020) This is an even bigger concern for kids with disabilities who attend First Nations schools, as their schools frequently cannot manage to provide them with the necessary resources and assistance (Derenisky, 2020).

POST-SECONDARY EDUCATION

University level education is a treaty right promised by Canada to Indigenous peoples. This was stated as a fundamental right in the 1982 Canadian Constitution Act ("First Nations, Inuit and Métis Education in Ontario," 2017). Despite the fact that education is a basic human right, the history of colonialism, residential schools, the systematic separation of Indigenous children from their families, and frequent racism against First Nations, Inuit, and Métis peoples have created substantial obstacles to gaining postsecondary education. Even though the government does indeed have a moral and legal obligation to provide access to education, most Indigenous people are unable to attend college or university due to financial constraints ("First Nations, Inuit and Métis Education in Ontario," 2017). The tremendous rise of the Indigenous population, along with rising demand for college or university attendance, has put further strain on financing available for Indigenous peoples to pursue post-secondary education.

ACCESS TO POST-SECONDARY EDUCATION

Over 16,000 First Nations, Inuit, and Métis students are enrolled in universities and colleges in Ontario. However, there remains a considerable educational achievement disparity in Ontario between the Indigenous and non-Indigenous populations. In regards to university degrees, 29.3% of the non-Indigenous population has one, whereas just 11.3% of the Indigenous population has one

("First Nations, Inuit and Métis Education in Ontario," 2017). There is no discernible difference in college-level accomplishment, where costs are typically one-third of those of universities. Indigenous peoples living on reserves are much less likely to have access to education. Almost half of the Indigenous population living on a reserve does not possess a high school diploma ("First Nations, Inuit and Métis Education in Ontario," 2017).

FUNDING FOR INDIGENOUS EDUCATION

Indigenous education funding was legally acknowledged as the federal government's role in 1956 as part of the commitment to respect the Constitution and signed Treaties from the 18th century. Indigenous and Northern Affairs Canada (INAC) is responsible for providing financing methods to assist Indigenous students in paying for the cost of post-secondary education ("First Nations, Inuit and Métis Education in Ontario," 2017). INAC now oversees the Post-Secondary Student Support Program (PSSSP), the University and College Entrance Preparation Program (UCEPP), the Post-Secondary Partnership Program (PSPP), as well as other workforce development, job experience, and vocational training initiatives ("First Nations, Inuit and Métis Education in Ontario," 2017). The PSSSP and UCEPP give financial assistance to qualified First Nations and Inuit students participating in postsecondary programs. Both programs assist students in advancing academically and improving employability for First Nations and Inuit students. The PSPP funds postsecondary institutions to provide courses for First Nations and Inuit students, along with course conception and delivery ("First Nations, Inuit and Métis Education in Ontario," 2017). The PSPP focuses on expenditures connected with particular tasks relating to First Nations and Inuit education instead of allocating capital funds or money directly to students.

The federal government solely assists First Nations and Inuit students financially. Métis students in Ontario can qualify for the Métis Student Bursary Program (MSBP), which is administered by the Métis Nation of Ontario and is accessible in 42 post-secondary schools across the province (MNO). The MSBP awarded 200 bursaries totalling $136,772 in 2015-2016 ("First Nations, Inuit and Métis Education in Ontario," 2017). The MNO works hard to establish and improve programs in order to provide greater opportunities for Métis students in postsecondary education. In Daniels v. Canada (Indigenous Affairs and Northern Development), the Supreme Court of Canada (SCC) declared on April 14, 2016, that Métis and non-status Indians have to be acknowledged as "Indians" under section 91(24) of the Canadian Constitution ("First Nations, Inuit and Métis Education in Ontario," 2017). Despite knowing that the federal government owes Métis and non-status Indians a fiduciary obligation, the government has failed to revise the PSSSP to accommodate these two groups. The Supreme Court has not required the federal government to adjust current laws and programs to reflect the Daniels decision's conclusions, but instead wants these communities to hold the federal government accountable for rectifying their historical disadvantage ("First Nations, Inuit and Métis Education in Ontario," 2017).

THE FUNDING GAP

The PSSSP offers financial assistance to First Nations and Inuit people that is handled regionally and is intended to pay for the costs of tuition, textbooks, supplies, transportation, and living expenses. Prior to 1992, it was anticipated that all qualifying students would get financial assistance. Rather than being decided by the number of qualified students, the PSSSP became a scheme that simply gave a portion of cash irrespective of student demand in 1992. By 1996, the federal government had set a two-percentage-point yearly ceiling on PSSSP budget increases, irrespective of how many students registered ("First Nations, Inuit and Métis Education in Ontario," 2017). Ever since, financing has lagged behind increases in student demand, living expenses, inflation, and tuition costs. The federal government's shortage of financing has led regions that administer the grants to make difficult judgments about who gets support each year. INAC provided financial aid to 22,000 status First Nations and Inuit students in 2014-2015; the amount remained the same in 2006 ("First Nations, Inuit and Métis Education in Ontario," 2017). Prior to the implementation of the budget restriction, however, around 27,000 students were given financial assistance. A shortage of federal financing was expected to have prevented around 22,500 persons from pursuing postsecondary education by 2007. The federal government's latest $90 million investment to the PSSSP program for 2 years is a fantastic move, but it does not address the growing Indigenous youth population or the risk for financing instability in the coming years ("First Nations, Inuit and Métis Education in Ontario," 2017). When a budget limit is in effect, communities may be certain that they will not get more than the amount authorised. When the current government commits 90 million dollars for 2 years, there is no guarantee that the funds will continue ("First Nations, Inuit and Métis Education in Ontario," 2017). As a result, Indigenous students face significant barriers to obtaining postsecondary education in Canada. Employers today demand some level of post-secondary education in a nation where getting a job is correlated with completing education beyond high school. Increasing First Nations graduation rates to levels equivalent to the Canadian population would result in a $401 billion (2006 Dollars) financial advantage and a $115 billion reduction in government expenditure. The Auditor General of Canada found in 2004 that closing the education gap between First Nations individuals living on reserve and the rest of the Canadian population might take 27 years ("First Nations, Inuit and Métis Education in Ontario," 2017). The deficit had not yet been closed, according to the Auditor General's 2011 progress report. There has not been a consistent approach to closing the gap premised on the 2004 recommendations, nor has the government completely adopted an implementation plan in accordance with the audit ("First Nations, Inuit and Métis Education in Ontario," 2017). While the PSSSP's influence is diminishing, non-status First Nations and Métis peoples are still completely excluded from federal laws governing Indigenous support. Because the PSSSP is inaccessible to these students, thousands are unable to enter a post-secondary university. In addition to raising PSSSP funding, there have been repeated proposals to expand eligibility to include non-status and Métis students ("First Nations, Inuit and Métis Education in Ontario," 2017).

Undergraduate tuition costs in Ontario have climbed by 248% since 1993-1994, making public universities unaffordable to a greater number of students. The Ontario government offers very little financing for Indigenous postsecondary education in the province. The provincial government contributed $5 million to the nine Indigenous institutions in 2015 ("First Nations, Inuit and Métis Education in Ontario," 2017). Excluding the Aboriginal Bursaries Search Tool, which was created in 2009, Indigenous students do not get direct financial help from the government. Ontario distributes $1.5 million in bursaries every year, which is insufficient for the 16,036 Indigenous students who attend college or university in the province. The majority of the provincial government's investment in Indigenous postsecondary education goes to colleges and universities for support programs, counsellors, curriculum, and teaching initiatives ("First Nations, Inuit and Métis Education in Ontario," 2017).

CHALLENGES TO PROGRESS

There is a fundamental divergence in the definition of education between Indigenous communities and the federal and provincial governments of Canada. Sovereignty, not subjection to another authority, is the beginning point for First Nations. As sovereigns, Indigenous people consider education as a broad notion, not one restricted to brick-and-mortar schools and K-12 schooling (Sékaly & Bazzi, 2021). For Indigenous People, the concept and delivery of education must be consistent with their culture, history, and customs. One of the most significant challenges confronting Indigenous people is governance or authority over educational decisions.

The Federal Government's traditional ethos of "knowing best" persists in many facets of everyday life in the Indigenous territory, impeding Indigenous communities' capacity to manage their own future (Sékaly & Bazzi, 2021). Inadequate line-item budgets that require Indigenous people to seek approval before reallocating funds from one school line to another impede the Indigenous community's capacity to fulfil local needs rapidly. An Indigenous tribe, for example, may have a larger proportion of pupils who require special education services. They should not require Ottawa's permission to reallocate funds from the overall education budget to address such needs.

The overall amount of education financing for Indigenous people is a substantial impediment to closing the learning gap, as evidenced in several reports and studies over the years. Indigenous communities will never be able to overcome the consequences of previous colonial activities and narrow the learning gap for their pupils unless suitable resources are provided. Aside from appropriate, continuous, and regular financing, there are a few essential building blocks that will be critical in ensuring that Indigenous children have equal access to excellent education and achieve comparable educational achievements as non-Indigenous children (Sékaly & Bazzi, 2021). Given the significance of Indigenous culture, it is critical that these schools have room for Elders who will be accessible to help pupils, as well as space for traditional and cultural activities. Given the likelihood that schools will also function as gathering places for Indigenous people, these structures should feature community-oriented spaces to act as a community hub (Sékaly & Bazzi, 2021).

The second important impediment is the lack of a comprehensive curriculum in the Indigenous people's language that reflects its culture, history, and customs. The Indigenous education system must support and guarantee that each Indigenous community's language, culture, history, arts, and abilities are passed down to the next generation and subsequent generations (Sékaly & Bazzi, 2021). This includes establishing and/or improving immersion programs in the language to reclaim lost ground. Each Indigenous community must have the freedom to spend the funds in the way that best suits its unique circumstances. In all circumstances, learning materials for all grades must be prepared, and the curriculum must emphasise each unique Indigenous community's culture and language.

To teach an Indigenous-centric curriculum, instructors must be proficient in the language as well as knowledgeable about the Indigenous people's culture and history. Qualified teachers are the bedrock upon which great education for Indigenous kids is built. In Canada, there are various faculties of education that provide specialties for Indigenous teachers (Sékaly & Bazzi, 2021). It is critical not just to recruit these teachers but it is also critical to keep them in the community. Indigenous schools, particularly in more rural areas, have struggled to attract and retain skilled instructors. When there was a teacher shortage, Indigenous communities were able to recruit younger instructors who were early in their careers and looking for teaching experience. After accumulating teaching experience, these instructors would be transferred to provincial systems. We are now entering a period of teacher shortage, with school districts competing for skilled instructors (Sékaly & Bazzi, 2021). This will make recruiting and retaining qualified teachers much more difficult. To help in the recruitment and retention of talented teachers, salary and benefits parity with the provincially financed system is required. Furthermore, extra incentives, particularly in more remote regions, may be required to realise the increased expenditures in those places. It is also critical to improve Indigenous people's access to teacher education. This may be accomplished through Indigenous institutes' courses and programs, as well as improved financial assistance (Sékaly & Bazzi, 2021). In certain circumstances, this may be the only method to locate a teacher who possesses cultural understanding and competence and who can be retained year after year.

The involvement of the community and the notion of "family-centred" education are two fundamental principles of Indigenous education (Sékaly & Bazzi, 2021). For Indigenous education to thrive, the historical burden of Indian education reform in Canada must be addressed. The social consequences of these government practices (residential schooling, forced assimilation, and language and culture loss) are still evident in Indigenous communities today. Specific services are required to help the school in effectively engaging with the community.

Furthermore, Indigenous people recognize the critical role of families in educational results, and that until the entire family is active and prospering, the individual student will not have the resources at home to thrive throughout their academic career. For the next generation of students to achieve, the legacy of previous government mistakes must be addressed. This can only be accomplished by ensuring that families have access to the necessary programs and services. This approach contrasts with the "student-centred focus" that is prevalent in many non-Indigenous institutions (Sékaly & Bazzi, 2021). Most parents want their children to be successful in their chosen fields. The emphasis on culture and language is intended to establish a firm foundation for learning.

STEPS TO CLOSE THE GAP

A few methods must be implemented in order to considerably reduce the educational learning gap between Indigenous students and non-Indigenous pupils in Canada. Many educational financing models allocate funds to local governments based on "inputs," which are financial amounts per unit of input (Sékaly & Bazzi, 2021). For example, $500 for learning materials per student. An outcome-based strategy must offer adequate funds to address structural performance inequalities, decades of underfunding, and deliberate actions by successive governments to degrade Indigenous language and culture. This outcome model would give each Indigenous community an overall educational budget, with each community making allocation decisions based on its particular circumstances, rather than being guided by a "central authority" on how to spend the resources. The Indigenous educational body would be held accountable to people of their community for how money is distributed and used, but more crucially, for student results. The fundamental principle is that the funding must be used for educational objectives as outlined by the Indigenous communities (Sékaly & Bazzi, 2021). To be able to take on this responsibility, Indigenous people may need to invest in increasing its capability. They are up to the task.

Accountability can be analogous to the accountability connection between the federal and provincial governments for medical transfers, or to the accountability relationship between provinces and municipalities (Sékaly & Bazzi, 2021). In addition to typical financial records, the Indigenous people might publish outcome-based reports on their students' educational progress.

The second proposal contends that Indigenous communities' full desires to offer a comprehensive approach to their children's education, which emphasises the crucial role of the community, must be acknowledged. Within that educational framework,

Indigenous communities must be given the authority and funding to create a curriculum that represents their language, culture, history, and educational philosophy (Sékaly & Bazzi, 2021). This entails fully integrating land-based education into classroom instruction. It also implies that Indigenous communities would create their own databases to assess their students' learning results. Because many Indigenous children attend high schools outside of their native region, the curriculum would have to follow the provincial curriculum (Sékaly & Bazzi, 2021). Furthermore, these students must acquire a provincial graduation diploma in order to participate in higher education or apprenticeships if they so wish.

Giving Indigenous people the freedom to direct their financial resources to areas of most need would enable them to attract and retain talented instructors. This is especially challenging in rural, fly-in communities. Some of these instructors may need to participate in a "immersion" program to re-acquaint themselves with Indigenous languages (Sékaly & Bazzi, 2021). Indigenous people must have the freedom to invest in professional development while also adequately compensating instructors.

CONCLUSION

The word "equity" in the context of educational attainment is commonly used in public education. Equity is frequently associated with equity of opportunity, equity of access (to schooling, technology, resources, and mental health), equity of result, equity of resources, and eventually reducing the achievement gap, which means equity in graduation and a future (Sékaly & Bazzi, 2021). In a knowledge-based economy, completing a post-secondary education gives the marketable skills and training required for job placement and higher pay. If skills are not adequately transmitted, dependency on government transfers will expand, as will the disparity in labour market participation and post-secondary graduation rate among Indigenous and non-Indigenous communities. To close the enormous education gap and remove financial constraints to postsecondary education, government support must be immediate and increased for Indigenous students in postsecondary education ("First Nations, Inuit and Métis

Education in Ontario," 2017). Students who are able to obtain government support and a college or university degree go on to become leaders in their respective fields and make significant contributions to their communities.

REFERENCES

Derenisky, K. (2020, August 19). Eliminating Educational and Employment Gaps. Kathryn's Teaching Journey. https://edusites.uregina.ca/kdereniskyeportfolio/?p=304

First Nations, Inuit and Métis Education in Ontario. (2017, January). Canadian Federation of Students–Ontario. https://www.cfsontario.ca/wp-content/uploads/2018/10/2017.01-Indigenous-Education-fact-sheet.pdf

Sékaly, G., & Bazzi, R. (2021, May 19). A Critical Perspective on the Canadian Education Gap: Assessing First Nation Student Education Outcomes in Canada. StrategyCorp. https://strategycorp.com/2021/05/assessing-first-nation-student-education-outcomes-in-ca nada/

CONCLUSION

Throughout the chapters, we have explored numerous topics. These incidents show how Canada's treatment of Indigenous peoples has been unfair. From a mutually respectful partnership, Wampum belts and residential institutions, these are examples of the events. Indigenous peoples voluntarily signed treaties, but as a result of these acts of vile discrimination, they were later subjected to. Even though there is a growing awareness of these injustices today, Indigenous Canadians continue to fight for the restoration of the past and the fulfilment of the promises made in treaties.

Instead of reacting reactively to the effects of Indigenous communities suffering from prolonged exposure to excessive environmental hazards placed within and near their lands, Canada must learn from its mistakes in the future and be able to address the health of Indigenous communities from a proactive and preventive standpoint.

The improvement of Canadian society as a whole, not just indigenous communities, depends on the healthcare system. It is time for Canadian society to recognise the injustice that exists in the way that native people are treated and to take prompt, effective corrective action.

The mental health of Indigenous people is worse than that of the non-indigenous population. Many things, including a lack of education, stigmatisation fears, a lack of resources and opportunity, may contribute to this. Therefore, developing measures to support the promotion of mental health in these communities is crucial. To support these groups, strategies including education promotion, stigma reduction, and policy introduction must be put into practise.

The jurisdictions imposed on their ancestors in the wake of the Indian Act of 1876 are to blame for many of the issues that Indigenous people in Canada today face, including disproportionately high rates of poverty, unemployment, overrepresentation in the welfare system, and substance abuse problems. Indigenous children who were removed from their families and prohibited from learning about their heritage during years of residential schools grew up to be people who understood very little about their heritage. They had fewer career prospects than their non-Indigenous counterparts due to the poor education they acquired at these institutions, which resulted in impoverishment for many survivors who ended themselves on the streets.

Indigenous people have a close bond with animals, which is a strong indication of how important this relationship is to them. Due to the long history of interdependence between animals and Indigenous people, animals now play a significant role in Indigenous culture (Weatherdon, 2022). Indigenous people have a close bond with the animals, which is why they treat them with respect. This relationship demonstrates how these two groups are very dependent on one another and play a significant part in one another's lives. Mutual respect and mutual benefit are the foundations of this relationship.

Allyship is difficult and lasts a lifetime. Going back to the idea of cultural humility, being an ally necessitates a dedication to being reflective and persistently seeking out new knowledge to better oneself. More authentic allyship can be cultivated by thinking about the growth of one's intersectional lens, taking part in workshops, reading materials written by Indigenous authors, and reflecting on one's own prejudices and presumptions.